HANDBOOK OF MILK MICROBIOLOGY

HANDBOOK OF
MILK MICROBIOLOGY

Manish L. Srivastava

2016
Daya Publishing House®
A Division of
Astral International Pvt. Ltd.
New Delhi - 110 002

© AUTHOR
First Impression, 2002
Reprinted, 2016

ISBN: 978-93-5124-381-6 (International Edition)

Published by : **Daya Publishing House®**
A Division of
Astral International Pvt. Ltd.
– ISO 9001:2008 Certified Company –
4760-61/23, Ansari Road, Darya Ganj
New Delhi-110 002
Ph. 011-43549197, 23278134
E-mail: info@astralint.com
Website: www.astralint.com

Laser Typesetting : **Classic Computer Services**
Delhi - 110 035

Digitally Printed at : **Replika Press Pvt. Ltd.**

TO
GOD SAI NATH

PREFACE

In writing this book we have tried to present an account of modern Milk Microbiology that is both through the accerrible since our subject is brad. Covering a diversity of topics from viruses to helminths (by way of the bacteria) and from patlogenicity to physical chemistry, this can make presentation of a coherent treatment difficult but it is also part of what makes food microbiology such on interesting and challenging subject.

This book is directed primarily at students of food microbiology and some related subjects up to master's level and assumer some knowledge of basic microbiology of milk. We have chosen not to burden the text with reference to the primary literature in order to preserve what we hope is a rearulble harrative flow. Some suggestions for further reading for each chapter are included.

Industrial microbiology encomparer abroad and complex area of study. It includes the many uses of microrganisms to produce products of economic value and to decompose the wastes of municipalities and industry. This book was write or an introductary text to produce the college junior and senior student or the industsrial technical heeling to gain on it sight into this area, with a working knowledge of the theory and practical of various aspects of milk microbiology.

Various concepts of industrial microbiology research also are considered in this book or are some of the techniques employed in the handling of industrial culturer, and in the dercion, array and purification of fermentation products. This text book in not intented primarily for those planning to pursure microbiology or their major field of in sterest nor for those industrials preparing for a carrer in milk. Because in Milk Microbiology Microber play or important role.

The references included suggested reading are necessarily restricted. Key review articles and books have been included, and in some cary, primary research reference which have becomes landmark. The biblography give in this literature covers all the references cited in the text.

Our thanks are to our many colleagues and students who were geneous with helpful community and spared their time for discussions, we would particularly like to thank ER. Mukundi Lal and Arima for his constant encouragement, help and valuable literature. We would also like to thank the personnel of the National Engineering Research Institute for help in several way, including providing literature.

We are particularly grateful Gurav and Santosh for guidance and in the source of several references. Finally we would like to thank Amit Lal to give suggestion and companiship during the period of writing.

We thanks Mr. Anil Mittal of Daya Publishing House for his cooperation in production of this book. Finally, we thank Mr. V.D. Upadhayay (Holland), Mrs. Samita Srivastava (Mexico), Dr. Smith (U.S.A.), Mr. Ankur Panda (Singapore), Dr. Monica Sinha (Germany), Dr. M. Parent (Japan), Dr. Jeannetle Navile (Canada) and Mansi Saxena (South Affrica) their help in numerous way and of this book.

M.L. SRIVASTAVA

CONTENTS

1

INTRODUCTION

Milk is the one of the complete foods which there seems to be no adequate substitute. All mammals produce milk after the birth of the young ones and man has used the milk of many animals as his food. Milk has good quality protein and the biological value is over 90. Though milk has good quality protein due to quality of protein and the amount that can be ingested and the presence of other nutrients makes is indispensable. India is essentially an agrarian country and bulk of its national income (Rs. 43,758 crores—1981-82) is derived from agricultural products. However, a considerable portion of this income originates from milk and milk products (totalling Rs. 73,00 crores). India's milk production now ranks first in Asia and third in the world (After U.S.S.R. and U.S.A.). With this huge production of milk, nearly 50 million tonnes per annum, the per capital consumption of milk is still below the recommendation of medical council of India (280 g/man/day), the reason being the huge human population of India. So, the following target was fixed for total milk production in the country (Table 1.1).

Milk is the fluid, excluding colostrum, secreated by mammals for the nourishment of their young. The principal components of milk are water, fat, protein and lactose.

Milk production may be fixed at any level. It will remain insufficient unless the human population of the country is kept under control. Although the production of milk is constantly increasing and per capita consumption is increasing as well, yet it is not reaching the level it is required.

In 1951 per capita of milk availability was 132, which is now 108 grams. On the other hand in 1966, it has increased to 163 grams. However, the regional and seasonal imbalance in our milk production do not permit this level of availability across the country. The sensitivity of the lean and flush characteristics of milk supply, with demand remaining constant the year-round, makes marketing of milk a real challenge. Milk production is insufficient is clear from the previous table. This inadequate amount of milk is not consumed in the form of fluid milk. There may be very many reasons for it. So some amount of fluid milk is converted into milk products.

Table 1.1
Total Milk Production in the Country

Year	Total Milk Production (Million Tonnes)	Per Capita Consumption (g/day)
1951	17.4	132
1956	19.7	135
1961	20.4	127
1966	19.4	108
1971-72	22.5	112
1977-78	28.3	123
1978-79	29.1	124
1979-80	30.2	126
1980-81	31.5	128
1981-82	32.9	131
1982-83	34.6	132
1983-84	36.3	135
1984-85	38.0	142
1986-87	44.0	156
1987-88	45.9	161
1988-89	50.0	163
1989-90 (Proj)	52.0	165
2000 – (Proj)	65.0	180

(Proj = Projected Value)

In India 50 per cent of the total milk production is utilized for making Indigenous milk products. Analysis of the latest available information indicated that India is producing nearly 100 million litres of milk per day. Generally the protein content of the milk reflects the growth rate of young animal—the higher the growth rate.

In 1976 National Commission on Agriculture has also projected the milk reqirement for AD 2000 in the following manner (Table 1.2).

Table 1.2
Milk Requirement for 2000 (million M.T.)

	Rural	Urban	Total
Low Estimate	31.81	17.55	49.36
High Estimate	42.39	22.01	64.40

It is apparent from Table 1.3 that only 54.5 per cent of milk production in the country is utilized as fluid milk and rest is converted into milk products (Western and Indigenous). Hence, the Indian Government affords are to increase milk production by improving breeding, feeding and better management and to procure maximum amount of fluid milk from production centres (villages) through co-operative societies. Lastly, to have check, on countrie's human population by family planning programme.

Table 1.3
Mode of Utilization

Mode of Utilization	Milk Utilized (Million litres/day)
1. Urban Scale	25.0
2. Proceed for distribution by dairy plants	5.0
3. Conversation into western dairy products	4.5
4. Conversation into Indigenous dairy products	50.0
5. Fluid milk in rural areas	15.5

Three sources contribute to the micro-organism found is milk the under interior, the teat exterior and its immediate surrounding and the milking and milk handling equipment. Milk can not be kept for a long period unless it is chilled or treated in one way or the other, because the growth of micro-organisation spoil milk and renders milk unfit for human consumption. Thus, the storage life of milk can be increased by converting it into various milk products, viz.—*Khoa, Ghee, Dahi,* Cheese, *Channa,* Ice cream etc. *Khoa* is a most common dehydrated milk product sold in the market. *Khoa* is hardly used as such in house hold or in market. It is always used as a base ingredient in the production of sweets such as *burfi*, *peda*, lodge etc. Cheese, *khoa* and dehydrated milk powder are concentrated froms hence contain high amounts per unit.

The market people (*halwai*) further increase self life of *khoa* by mixing sugar (locally knows as *boora*) to it. Thus, addition of *Boora* to *khoa* further increases its self life and also improve its taste. The *khoa* based sweets become more popular in the market. They are mostly prepared by untrained and illiterate *Halwais* moreover there is no standard technology for the preparation of these product hence day to day variation is always possible and found. Sometimes we except the variation of extreme nature not only this the way it is sold on the *halwai* shops is another serious problem, they are always sold on *halwai* shop in see these sweets. So sometimes, they are displayed in showcases and sometime in open pans. This result in a constant deterioration of sweets microbiologically.

Milk-handling equipments such as teat cups, pipework, milk holders and storage tanks are the principal source of the microorganism found in raw milk. Milk secretion of mammary glands of mammals is complete food. Freshly drawn milk greatly varies in chemical composition depending on its source and status of animal health. Milk contains vitamins A, B_1, and B_2. It contains small amounts of vitamin C and D besides, smaller quantities of other vitamins. Lysine is one of the essential amino acid which is abundant in milk proteins.

1. MICROFLORA OF MILK

The sources contribute to the micro-organism found in milk the under interior, the teat exterior and its immediate surroundings, and the milking and milking handling equipment. There are several principal sources of contamination of milk, from the time milk leaves the udder, until it is transferred to containers, everything with which it comes in contact as a potential source of contribution of micro-organisms. Milking performed under hygienic conditions with strict attention to sanitary practices, will reduce the entry of micro-organisms in the milk. Milk when kept raw, contain more number of micro-organisms than the boiled milk. Generally *Lactobacillus*, *Streptocoocus*, *Micrococci*, *Coliform* and Spore formers are present in large numbers.

The rate at which organisms increase in milk is determined primarily by two factors—temperature of holding and species present therein.

The holding temperature also greatly influences the types of organisms that grow, since the maximum, optimum and minimum growth temperature vary widely with different species.

Milk secreted by the udders of a healthy cow is sterile, but it frequently gets contaminated at the time it is drawn from the animal. The number of micro-organisms contained when milk leaves the stable vary from a few thousand per milliliter or even less than 1000 under controlled methods of production to 50,000 or more per unit.

The types of micro-organisms found in milk vary considerably and are dependent upon the specific conditions associated with the batch of the milk. Bacteria, yeast, moulds and bacteriophages are commonly encountered. In milk and milk products, viruses and protozoa are seldom observed, except as occasional contaminants.

Bacteria

Bacteria are the most common and probably the most numerous of micro-organisms with which the dairy processing industry is concerned. They belong to four main groups (i) Cocci (ii) Gram positive non-sapor forming rods (iii) gram positive spore forming rods and (iv) gram negative non-sporeforming rods.

Yeast

The yeast most frequently encountered in milk and milk products act upon the lactous to produce acid and CO_2.

Moulds

Moulds often grow in large concentrations and are visible as a furry or fluffy growth. They are black, gray, green, blue or white.

Bacteriophages

They are particularly obnoxious in starter cultures.

Table 1.4
Estimated Number of Microbes in Milk

Point of sampling	Usual range
Asseptically drawn milk	500-1000
Milk pail	1000-10,000
Bulk milk tank	5,000-20,000

2. SOURCE OF CONTAMINATION

There are several principal sources of contamination of milk. From the time milk leaves the udder, until it is dispensed in containers, everything with which it comes in contact is a potential source of micro-organisms.

Milking performed under hygienic conditions, will reduce the entry of micro-organisms in the milk. Sources of micro-organisms are :

1. The producing animal

Unless the producing animal is clean and her flanks, udder and teats given special sanitary care just before milking, her body can be a source of considerable contamination. The first few streams of milk from each test should be discarded. Milk from an infected animal is likely to contain a large number of microbes. The probability of diseases of the udder contaminating the milk is very high.

2. The milking area

The microbial content of air is greatly affected by many conditions and practices. Dried dirt and filth is picked up by air movements and carried about as dust in the atmosphere. For this reason, dust may be a source of almost every kind of contamination.

3. Utensils and equipments

These items are known to be greatest sources of contamination. These may account for as much as 1,00,000 to a billion organisms per millilitre. Pails, stainer, milking machines, cans, pipes, bottles and other equipments used for the handling of milk are sometimes not properly washed and sanitized. Organisms survive in cracks, crevices and other irregularities of the utensils.

4. Personnel

All persons involved in milking process must be in good health and must be careful in their personal cleanliness. They should wash their hands, clean and rinse them with an effective bacteriological solution. A surgical mask is an effective addition to the uniform.

5. Water

Water is continuously required for cleaning and processing operation in a diary, the microbiological quantity of water is tested before it is used in a dairy plant. The most common test for water destined for domestic or industrial use is presumptive coliform test. Chlorination of water is commonly practiced to assure potability.

There are two main sources of contamination :

On the Farm : Milk contains relatively few bacteria when it leaves the udder of a healthy cow and generally these bacteria do not grow in milk under the usual conditions of handling. During normal milking operation; however milk is subject to contamination from the animal, especially the exterior of the udder and adjacent areas. Bacteria found in manure, soil and water may enter from this source. Fewer organisms enter this way when a milking machine is used than, when milking is done by hand. Such contamination can be reduced by clipping the cow and washing the udder with water or a germicidal solution before milking.

Probably the wo most significant sources of contamination are dairy utensils and milk contact surfaces, surface including the milk pail or milking machines and the bulk milk cooler. If dairy utensils of the milk contact surfaces are inadequately cleaned, sterilized and dried, bacteria may develop in large number in the dilute milk like residue and enter the next milk to touch these surface. Undesirable bacteria from these sources include lactic *Streptococci, Coliform bacteria* and *Thermodurics,* those which survive pasteurization.

Other possible sources of contamination are the hands and arms of the milker or dairy workers, the air of the barn and flies.

At manufacturing level: Other sources of contamination the milk leaves the farm includes the tanker truck, transfer pipes. The paper stock or the glass bottles used for packaging fluid milk are also an important source of contamination.

3. SPOILAGE OF MILK

Milk is an excellent culture medium for many kinds of micro-organisms, being high in moisture, nearly neutral in pH and rich in microbial foods. A plentiful supply of food for energy is present in the form of milk sugar, butterfat, citrate and nitrogenous compounds in many forms, besisdes as accessory food and minerals required by micro-organisms. Some inhabitory substance are present in freshly drawn milk but soon become ineffective. Because of fermentable sugar; an acid fermentation by bacteria is most likely under ordinary conditions in raw milk, but other changes may take place, if conditions are unfavourablee to the acid formers or if they are absent.

When milk sours, it usually is considered spoiled, especially if it curdles although the lactic and fermentation of milk is utilized in the manufacture of fermented milks and cheese. In raw milk at temperature from 10 to 37°C *Streptococcus lactis* is most likely to cause the souring with possibly some growth of *Coliform* bacteria.

The pasteurization of milk kills the more active acid-forming bacteria but they permits the survival of heat-resistant lactics which will cause lactic acid formation at higher temperature. The various ways of spoilage are:

Gas Production : Gas production by bacteria usually is accompanied by acid formation in milk. The chief gas formers are the *Coliform* bacteria, *Clostridium* spp. and gas forming Bacilli that yield both hydrogen and CO_2. The production of gas in milk is evidenced by foam at the top.

The likelihood of gas formation and type of mirco-organism causing it depend upon the pretreatment of the milk and the temperature of holding. In raw milk the coliform bacteria are most apt to be the main gas formers. Gas forming *Clostridium* and *Bacillus* do not compete well with acid formers at higher temperature but may function if the acid formers are absent.

Proteolysis : The hydrolysis of milk proteins by micro-organisms usually is accompanied by the production of bitter flavour caused by some peptides released. Proteolysis is favored by storage at low temperature.

The type of change produced by proteolytic micro-organisms include; (1) Acid proteolysis, in which acid production and proteolysis occur together; (2) Proteolysis with little acidity or even with alkalinity; (3) Sweet curdling which is caused by renin like enzymes of the bacteria at an early stage of proteolysis; (4) Slow proteolysis and (5) Residual proteolysis.

Acid proteolysis causes the production of shrunken curd. Actively proteolytic bacteria are found among the species of *Micrococcus, Pseudomonas, Flavobacterium* etc.

Ropiness : Ropiness or aliminess occur in milk due to :

1. Stringness caused by mastitis.
2. Sliminess resulting from the thickness of cream.
3. Stringness due to this films of caesin.

Bacterial ropiness is caused by slimy capsular material from the cells. There are two main types of bacterial ropiness, one in which milk is most ropy at the top and other in which milk becomes ropy throughout. Surface ropiness is caused by *Alcaligenes viscolactis.*

Changes in Milk Fat : Milk fat may be decomposed by various bacteria, yeasts and moulds, e.g. *Pseudomonas, Proteus, Bacillus.*

Alkali Production : The group of alkali formers include bacteria which cause an alkaline reaction in milk without any evidence of proteolysis. Alkali formers are *Pseudomonas flurescens*.

Flavour Change : Some of the off flavours are :

Sour Flavor : Acidity may be produced by *Streptococcus lactis* and *Leuconóstoc*.

Bitter Flavour : Bitterness usually results from proteolysis but may follow lipolysis or even fermentation of lactose. Milk from cows late in lactation period sometimes is slightly bitter.

Burnt Flavour : Certain attains of *Streptococcus lactis* produces this flavour, which resembles the overheated milk.

Colour Changes : The colour changes are :

Blue milk - *Pseudomonas syncyanea* produced a bluish gray to brownish colour in milk in pure culture but when growing with an acid former like *Streptococcus lactis* causes a deep blue colour.

Yellow milk - *Pseudomonas sysnxantha* may cause a yellow colour in the cream layer of the milk.

Red milk - Red milk usually is caused by species of *Serratia*.

Brown milk - A brown colour may result from *Pseudomonas putrefaciens*.

4. PRESERVATION OF MILK

Milk is such a delicately flavoured, easily perishable food that all sorts of preservatives cannot be used without causing an undesirable change in its taste, flavour and nutritional value. There are specific methods that are employed for its preservation.

Asepsis : Prevention is the best method. Keeping quality is usually improved when smaller number of micro-organisms are present. The exterior of the cow and milk contact swurfaces have been emphasized as possible sources of both a high number and undesirable kind of microbes, so aspetic conditions are most important. Packaging serves to keep microbes away from bottled milk.

Removal of micro-organisms

Use of Heat

Pasteurization and ultrapasteurisation : The milk heat treatment is called pasteurization. Objectives of pasteurization is; (1) To kill all the pathogens that may enter the milk and may be transmitted to people; (2) To improve the keeping quality of milk. Ideally this heat treatment should be accompanied without deleteriously affecting the flavour, appearance, nutritional properties and cream value of the milk.

The first widely used pasteurization process for milk involved heating the milk in large tanks or vats to 60°C for at least 20 minutes. This holding method was subsequently changed to 61.7°C for 30 min and finally to 62.8°C for 30 min, to eliminate *Coxiella burnetii*. This process is called vat pasteurization (HTST) system. Heat treatment process in excess of pasteurization for milk and products have designated as very-high temperature (VHT) systems and ultra high temperature (UHT) system. UHT processes usually refer to pasteurization techniques with temperature at least 130°C in a continuous flow with holding times approximately 1 sec or more.

The efficiency of milk pasteurization or the percentage of reduction of numbr of microbes in milk during pasteurization depends upon:

(i)   The temperature of pasteurization
(ii) The holding time
(iii) The total number of bacteria
(iv) The proportion of total microbial load that are spore formers.

In general the conventional HTST system may reduce the number of micro-organisms in milk by at least 90 to 99%. Following pasteurization milk is cooled rapidly to at least 7.2°C or less.

Commercial pasteurization should kill all yeasts and moulds and most vegetative cells of bacteria in the milk. The surviving bacteria are the thermodurics.

Boiling : Boiling milk or heating in flowing steam destroys all micro-organisms except the spores of bacteria but changes the appearance and its digestibility.

Steam Under Pressure : Evaporated milk is canned and then heat processed by steam under pressure often with accompanying rolling or agitation. The forewarming of the milk at about 93 to 100°C or higher before evaporation kills all but the more resistant bacterial spores.

Use of Low Temperature

Refrigerated storage : For the production of milk of good quality it is essential that it is cooled promptly after it is withdrawn from the cow. Milk is heat at refrigeration temperature during storage on the farm, in the truck or tank during transportation to plant or receiving station and during storage there.

Use of Preservatives

Added preservatives : The addition of preservatives is one of the methods for preservation. The use of serbic or propionic acid or one of their salts is permitted in cottage cheese, yogurt and processed cheese. The primary objective in adding a preservative to hard cheese is to prevent the surface growth of moulds and to increase its shelf life.

Added sugar acts as a preservative of sweetened condensed milk, it reduces the number of microbes. Sodium Chloride is also used as a preservative. The addition of formalin and hydrogen peroxide is also done.

So milk, when sterile, is quite good but when it contains large number of disease causing microbes it can be harmful also. Therefore contamination of milk must be decreased by :

1. Aseptic conditions.
2. Utensils should be sterile.
3. Udders should be washed properly and regularly.
4. The health of the animal is also important.
5. All persons involved in milking process should be in good health.

6. Water used in cleaning and processing operation should be tested.

Thus, it is clear that the contamination of milk can be decreased just by taking some preventive measures. Therefore, this problem was selected as to know that upto what extent the number of micro-organisms are found in the milk samples from different dairies milk in the same city and that what is the effect of boiling the milk and keep in it at room temperature. As in rural areas the people are not much educated and they do not know what sanitary measures can be taken. So, in villages many diseases are caused just by mere contamination of milk due to and lack of education and lack of maintenance of proper hygenic conditions.

In this problem the primary aim was to know that what in the difference in milk obtained from different dairies and vendors, because in every place the source of contamination may be different, so to know the sources of contamination and also to. find out the difference in the number of micro-organisms in boiled and raw milk would serve a basic purpose in improving the milk. In boiled milk the micro-organisms are decreased at a high percentage than raw milk. Thus, the problem was selected to work on these basic data and so that we can educate people about the sources of contamination, the micro-organisms found in milk and the disease caused by them and also how to keep the milk fresh and free from micro-organisms for a longer time. By this we can help people to cope up with diseases caused by milk contamination. However, this is a very preliminary study in this field and much scope of work remains ahead.

2

FOOD MICROBIOLOGY

The human being have a widespread nutritional requirements their most of micro-organism. Human diet includes a variety of substances from many sources. The microbes are important part of our environment. They are ubiquitous and even the food material we are use is often associated with a number of microbes. Our food contains a variety of nutrients which is sufficient for growth of microbes also. Thus, food serves as an excellent media for microbes. The food microbes produces undesirable changes and renders the food unsafe for use. The contamination may originated from search of origin, harvesting/slaughter, processing, Transportation and storage etc. It was estimated that as much as 1/3 of world food supply was spoiled by microbes. In certain microbes are added to the food materials to produce a desirable change in it and to get specific products, so, flavors and texture of food is improved in some cases due to microbial activity. Hence, food microbiology is important field of study major aims of food microbiology.

1. Preservation of food by eliminating microbes responsible for its spoilage and deterioration.
2. The detection and preservation of food poisoning due to pathogenic micro-organisms.
3. Application of microbes to produce new foods and to preserve and improve their desirable characteristics.

Food Safety

Food has been having a long associates with transmission of disease. Regulation governing food hygiene can be found in early sources as old Testament, and writings of Confusims, Hinduism and Islam. Even today, food borneillness is pernaps most widespread health problems and important causes of reduced economic productivity (W.H.O., 1992). Evidences clearly indicates that biological contaminants are the major cause. Hence, food safety is an important part of food microbiology.

Initial contamination of fresh food. A variety of food and food product are used by man and other animals. Eight main division of food are important: Cereal and cereal products. All of these can broadly be classified as plant and Animals products. Another Classification of food can be basis of stability.

1. Perishable food like meat and fish.
2. Semi-perishable floods like potatoes.
3. Stable foods like cereals, flew and sugar.

But under moist condition, the stable or semi-perishable food becomes perishable.

A. *Plants products:* Usually the internal tissues of whole, healthy plant tissues or fruit are sterile, i.e. free from microbes however, external surface of there products are contaminated by microbes from different sources i.e.: soil, air, insects, handling by human, and improves packing. The magnitude of this microbial contamination reflects one or more of the following: - Environment from which food was taken: condition of raw product, method of handling, and time and condition of storage, High microbial count suggests that same undesired event has occurred and food is unfit for consumption.

The plant products provides a considerable past of human food specially in our country. Almost every part of plant, stem, root, flowers, fruits and tubers and leaves etc. are used for food. Although plants have evolved many mechanism to present microbial immersion of their tissues. Surfaces have a durable cuticle; gaseous exchange only though specialized openings, plant tissues have the antimicrobial agents, frequently phenolic metabolites, complex poly phenolic polymer called lignin, which is resistent to microbes. Many plants produce complex antimicrobial polymers, phytoalexins: which are resistant. The contamination of important plant products can be desired as:-

1. *Contamination of cereals and cereal products:* They are most important part of food: belong to Graminae: e.g. *Tritcum aestimum, T. dusam, Zea mays, Oryza sativa, Sorghum Vulgare* etc. The exteriors of harvested Grains have natural flora while growing and contamination from soil and water etc. Freshly harvested Grain have thousand for bacteria/g and spores of smuts and rusts Bacteria are mostly of families Pseudomonadaceae, Micrococeaceae, Lactobacillaceae and Bacillaceae. The field fungi includes *Fusarium culmerum, F. graminearum, Alternaria alternata, Chadesporium hesbarum* while these appears during improper storage of Grain are Alternaria, Fusarium and Penicillium.

2. *Contamination of Sugars and Sugar products:* They are low in moisture high osmotic pressure a prevented microbial growth but when diluted, decomposed are easily. The raw juice from sucrose is highly contaminated microbes are slime produces, e.g. sps of *leuconestoe* and Bacillus, genera of micrococcus, flavobacterium, Azbromobacters, yeast like saccharomyces, candida etc., a few moulds come from improbes handing in mills; 3600- 5×10^8/ml contamination may came from debris a fine particles on side or joints of trough of plants various process up to classification of sugars, reduces number of microbes in final product.

   The maple syrup is sterile in vascular bundles but contaminated from out side in tap holder, spout, plastic tecbing, and their equipments. A number of yeast and bacteria presents.

   Honey is contaminated by nectar and honey bees. A variety of yeasts may be present. Candies in market have up to 2×10^6/ piece of bacteria originating from air dust and handling.

3. *Contamination of vegetables and vegetable products:* The root caps, carrots and beets are covered by soil microbes, but these are relatively stable unless spoiled or cells are damaged. The low growing leafy vegetables like spinae, cabbage and letterce are heavily contaminated. The products have softer surface and easily imaded by microbes from time of harvesting and transporting upon

reach of consumers, they are contaminated by variety of microbes from time of harvesting and transporting up to reach of consumers, they are contaminated by variety of microbes like pecxtinolytic bacteria on leafy vegetables. Soil is also important field source of contaminated. The spoiled vegetables can spread contamination to fresh ones. Pathogens like salmonella and shigella from faces of birds and animals. *Clostridium botualium*, natural reservoir in soil may also be present, various fungi like botrytis (on may plants), *Tricothecium* rescus (Tomato, cauerpits), Fusarium coesulam (potato) are also accuse of a number of diseases plants, also *Aspergilus, baertilce Streptomyces, Pseudomonas, corynebacterium*, etc. from soil, water and handling sources, and infected plants.

4. *Contamination of fruits and fruit products:* Fruits grow same level at are grand; mainly contaminated by microbes of insects and by air microbes. Air microbes are principally soil microbes. Fruits also have high, sugars content and same what acidic. Thus, likely to be decomposed by yeasts (grapes) and moulds (citrus fruits). Also contaminated by improves handling and storing equipments. The penicillium digitcetum and digitatum on citrus fruit as comycetes like Monilinia may also be present on fruits. Grey mould, botrytis cinerice involved in spoilage of strawberries etc.

5. *Contamination of pulses Nuts and oil seeds:* Belongs to leguminaceae, paplionaceae and fabaceous, rich serve of protein contaminated from soil in fields, water of irrigation, air microflora etc. A number of moulds present *Aspergillus nigar, A. tomerii, Rhizopus*, Penicillium etc. may also be contaminated during harvesting etc.

B. *Contamination of Animal products:* As plant products, the animal products are likely to be contaminated by environmental and human factors:

1. *Contaminated of Meat and Meat products:* The internal portion of meat is free from microbes if a healthy animal is properly slaughtered; as in abattoir by a below on head, or by cutting the juggler vein, but it gets immediately

contaminated on exposure in abattoir some microbes can be defined from hides, hairs, gastrin testival, skin etc. During bleeding handling and using various microbes from gloves, equipment's etc. may contaminate the meat products. The frozen meats generally only have normal microbial flora from surfaces due to environment only. Exterior of animal harbeurs large number of microbes as from soil, water, feed and manure natural surface flora. The contaminated also raised from storage equipments like caner, boxes etc. Among the most common bacteria on fresh meats the *staphylo cocci*, micrococci, Enterococci and coliforms are common the low temperature. Preservation of meats famous psychrophilic micro-organism, e.g. Moraxela (Non-formentive, graminae roots). *Enterobacter, serratia*, Pseudomonas sps; cornobacterium, leuconostoc etc. are also associates with meats. Sps. of fungi includes Cladosporium, penicillium, mucor Alternaria, yeasts, minutia etc. can also be responsible for contamination of meet and its products. To maintain the quality of meats various of techniques (e.g. cold cells) and standard adapted to minimize microbes contents.

2. *Contamination of poultry products:* The freshly dressed eviscerated poultry have a bacterial flora on the surface that originates from bacteria normally present on the live birds and the manipulation during killing, defeathering and evisceration. Under good sanitary condition, bacterial count is 100-1000/cm^2 of skin, but under unhygienic condition, it is about hundred times or more. The intestinal flora of birds adds during evisceration microbes involved are *pseudomonas achrenobacter* Flavobacterium, micro coccus, coliform and yeasts like Torulopsis, trichorporon, candida, Rhodotorule etc.

3. *Contamination of eggs:* The interior of freshly laid egg is usually free from microbes. It is subsequent microbial content is determined by sanitary conditions under which it is held, as well as condition of storage like temperature and humidity. The shells of egg may soon be contaminated by faecal matter from hen, by living of nest by wash water eggs are washed, by handling and perhaps material in which eggs are packed. The bacteria and

moulds enters eggs through cracks in shells or when the bloom, (thin protein coats) covering the shall deteriorates. As eggs are kept at low temperate, low temperature bacteria like pseudomonas, protein achnomobacter, alcaligener, flanobacterium, micrococcus, coliform bacteria and moulds are most prevalent. Most of bacteria are Gram positive cocci or rods. Salmonella may be present on shall or in the shall or laid build up during processing etc.

4. *Contamination of Fishes:* The microbial flora of freshly caught sigh reveals quality of waters from which it is caught. The slime covering water surface of fish contains bacteria *Pseudomonas, Achrmobacter, Micrococcous, Serratia, Vibrio,* and bacillus, fresh water fished also. Bacteria of Genera *Acromonas,* Leutobacillus, *Alcaligens* and *streptococcous.* The bacteria found in intestine are *Achremobacter, Pseudomonas, Flavobacterium, vibrio, Bacillus, clestridium, E. coli* etc. Bacteria on slims ranges from 100 to several million/cm^2.

The main importance lies whether water in sewage polluted is net. Because it may transmit a number of pathogen, i.e. human also. The sea food, like shell fish (crustaeenum and mollus) finfish etc. may have Vibrio parahaemolytion which spread various gastrointestinal epidemics in U.S. commonly found in Atlantic, pacific gulf coastal water etc. The shall fish growing contaminated H_2O_5 may be infected by virus and source of Hepatitis infection.

5. Milk and milk products: See milk microbiology.

Microbial spoilage of foods

What is spoilage: The real linguistic meaning of food spoilage is "deprive of good or effective qualities". In spoilage of food, it means that it is no more imputable due to some undesirable changes in it. In may be due to insect damage, drying out, discolouration, staling or rancidity and due to changes brought by micro-organisms word spoilage is also subjective, it is not necessary that food acceptable by one person(s) is also accepted by other(s). A general feature of microbial spoilage is relatively sudden onset: it does not appears to develop gradually, indicating that microbes can metabolize and grow at exponential rate.

Fitness or non-fitness of food for consumption

Although this criteria differs from person to person due to his choice accordingly, but some pts in judgement are common for fitness:

1. The desired stage of development or maturity: As fruits should be at a certain but differing stage of maturity (ripeness): sweet corn should be young birds preferred to be tended and milky: poultry from young bird preferred.

2. Freedom from contamination at any stage of production or handling: e.g. raw vegetables fertilized with sewage should be washed properly; tough effected by files or rodents is suspected.

3. Freedom from objection able changes resulting from microbial attack or action of enzymes of food but here, it is difficult to differ but desirable and undesirable change e.g. Putrefaction means spoilage but the process is common in ripening of Limberger cheese.

Major causes of food spoilage

1. Growth and activity of micro-organism (or higher forms occasionally), often a of organism is involved.
2. Insects.
3. Action of enzyme of plant or animal food.
4. Purely chemical reactions, i.e., these not catalyzed by enzymes of tissues or of micro-organisms.
5. Physical changes like freezing, drying, burning, pressure etc. According to the case of spoilage, food can be classified as perishable (meat, fish, poultry, dairy products etc.); Semi-perishable (potatoes, apples nut meats etc.) or Non-perishable (arch, sugars and dry beam etc.).

Microbial spoilage of foods

It is apparent that these is great variety of foods, hence, almost all microbes are potential contaminants. The type of food contents and the method by which it is processed or handled many farm mars certain groups of microbes in it, food is a good media for growth of microbes. It allowed to grow, organisms produce undesirable odious flavour and other qualities of food. The type of microbes that can grow and type and nature of spoilage are determined by following two factors:

1. The chemical properties of food product.
2. The method of processing and preservation.

A. Effect of chemical properties on spoilage: The chemical properties of food product influence the type of microbes that changes and hence determines the changes in appearance, odious flavour etc.

Composition of food: The nutrients present in food are most determining factor of microbial growth and spoilage carbohydrates are responsible for energy giving food. They are most common source of energy and food.

Complex carbohydrates like cellulose is utilised relatively by favour number of microbes. These are particularly hydrolyzed by yeast and moulds and fermentation takes place. The bacteria of genera *streptococcous, Leucomestoc* and *micrococcous* are *saccharolytic* and also can attack carbohydrates. The ability of same bacteria and moulds to hydrolyze 'pectin' results in softening or rotting of fruits and vegetables.

That facts are attacked by relatively low number of microbes only when more readily usable source, the sugars are absent. Mainly by moulds and a few Gram negative bacteria. They are hydrolyzed with help of lipase into glyecrol and fatty acids, which are then used by microbes. The fats undergo hydrolytic decomposition and become suncid as malodorous fatty acids are set free.

Protein are the food products used for growth of body. The microbes differs in their ability to use various nitrogenous compounds as a source of N_2. Some can hydrolyze proteins and others not hydrolysis of protein results in peptides, amino acids, NH_3 etc. which may be usable to one microbes and not to other. Usually many kinds of moulds are proteolytic but only a few bacteria and yeasts are actively proteolytic, bacteria sps. especially spose formers gram negative rods like pseudomonas and bacillus are proteolytic, few cocci can also attack proteins.

The accessory food substances are vitamins. Some microbes are unable to manufacture few of them. Hence, are derived from food stuffs itself. Egg white contains biotin but also contains avidin. Which ties it up making it unavailable to microbes and eliminating these which most have biotin supplied as possible spoilage organism.

Purification

Protein + Proteolytic microbes → Amino acids + Amines + NH_3 + Hydrogen sulphits

Fermentation

Carbohydrates + Carbohydrates → Acid + alcohol + Gases

Rancidity

Fatty foods + lipolytic microbes → Fattry acid + glycerol

The **appx** composition of different types of food given later.

Effect of Acidity or pH or Hydrogen ion concentration: It is important for the kinds of microbes that grow and type of spoilage that it produces. The reaction of nearly all foods is below pH 7.0. Foods are classified as Acid or new acid. The reaction of acid food is below pH 4.5 and that of new acid food is above pH 4.5 mostly fruits are acid foods while nearly all vegetables, fish, meat and milk products are man acids. In general bacteria grows fastest in pH ranges 6-8, yeasts 4.5-6.0, and filamentous fungi at 3.5-4.0. But there may be some exceptio also, e.g. Lactobacillus and acetic acid bacteria are acid produces and requires pH of about 5-6. Acid foods have low pH and thus, prevents growth of most of bacteria. They are spoilage by mainly yeasts and moulds. The vegetables, having moderately acid pH and soft rot producing bacteria like *Ercoinia carofanora* and *pseudomonas* plays a important role in their spoilage. Non-acids foods are likely to be spoiled by bacteria, but also supports growth of moulds under proper conditions.

The buffers are important in resist of pH changes and especially within specific pH ranges. Vegetable juice have low buffering power, so decrease of pH by only little lactic acid production by lactobacillus, thus facilitating rapid sulersiol microbes. Milk has high buffering power, permits considerable growth and acid production before growth of microbes is stopped and important for production of fermented milks.

Some inhibitory substances, added, accidently added or natural allows specific microbes to grow, e.g. lysozyme in egg white (natural); propionate brosorbic acid added to bread (to prevent ropiness, added); and treatment of processing equipment with insecticides, herbicides or detergents (accidently added) e.g. Propionic acid by propionic acid bacteria in Swiss cheese inhibits moulds.

The application of low pH is now a days employed a inhibitory effect on microbial growth by addition of weak organic acid.

A. Physical state and structure of food: Moisture and osmotic pressure = The growth of microbes requires at least 13% of free water in the foods. Moulds requires least free water and bacteria requires greatest free water. The moisture available also "must be available" for microbes is not tied up away in anyway, by solutes or by hydrophilic colloids like agar. Food with higher sugar and salt concentrations inhibits growth of microbes. Bacteria are inhibited by 3-15% of salt, but some moulds and yeast can tolerate up to 15% salt, 65-75% of sugar is required to inhibit moulds, while 50% for bacteria and most yeast. Foods of higher sugar or salt concentration are likely to be spoiled by moulds.

A useful parameter to understand movement of water bacteria environment and cytoplasm is water activity (a_w). It is defined as the ratio of partial pressure of water in the atmosphere in equilibrium with substrate B compared with partial pressure of atmosphere in equilibrium with pure water at same temperature (P_o).

Hence, moisture content and osmotic pressure is important for determining factor for types of microbes and spoilage.

$$a_w = \frac{P}{P_0} = \frac{1}{100} \text{ ERH (Equilibrium relative humidity)}$$

B. Effect of storage condition on spoilage of food: The presence of oxygen also determines types of microbes that grows and spoilage, e.g. Moulds and Aerobic bacteria grows only when a plenty of oxygen is available to them. Moulds are aerobic, most yeast grows best aerobically and bacteria of different kinds may be aerobic, anaerobic or facultative. The yeast and facultative bacteria can grow in closed containers as well as when exposed to the air. But *Clostridium* and other types can spoil food only under strict anaerobic conditions.

During limited oxygen, carbohydrates are oxidized by certain microbes into incomplete products like organ is acid, while in presence of oxygen, carbon dioxide and water are the product. The decomposition of proteins under anaerobic conditions results in putrefaction. The meat could support slime forming aerobic, souring bacteria at surface, or anaerobic types in its interior.

On the basis of O_2 requirement, the inhibitory effect of O_2 absence (supplied with CO_2) is used for preservation of a number of food commodities 50% for bacteria and most yeasts. Foods or higher sugar or salt concentrations are likely to be spoiled by moulds. A useful parameter to understand merement of water bet. Environment and cytoplasm is water activity (a_w). It is defined as the ratio of partial pressure of H_2O in the atmosphere in equilibrium with substrate P_0 compared with partial pressure of atmosphere in equilibrium with pure H_2O at same temperature, P_0.

MICROBIOLOGICAL EXAMINATION OF FOODS

The microbial examination of food products is very important from public health point of view and provides us with following informations:

1. The quality of raw food.
2. Sanitary condition under which food was processed.
3. Effectiveness of method of preservation of food.

It is possible to identify the agent responsible for spoilage and thus it is possible to trace source of contamination and conditions which permits the spoilage to occurs. Then temps are taken to prevent such spoilage. The practical procedure adopted depenɗs upon type of food and type of organism(s) to be traced. The objectives of microbiological tests will also depends upon type of agencies performing it. The purpose of Govt. labs is ascertain the standards of foods as governed by law, e.g. for Total bacterial count.

The food-plant laboratories, concerned with quality control test raw products and in gradients and hence, predicting type of problems that may arises and also, to met quality of products.

Private agencies might have lab tests to enable the recommendation of certain brands of foods. Commercial central agencies like America Dry milk institute set their own standards and recommends official method of examination.

1. Use of indicator organisms for microbial examination: Though general methods of examination of foods, but pathogen present in small amounts difficult to be examined. Alternative method is to look for an emaciated organism present in large number's i.e. indicator organism. A good indicator organism should always be present in large numbers when pathogen is present, it should not prediferate in environment being monitored.

E. coli is normal componert of Gut flora and implies same history of contamination from faecal origin. However limitations arises as presence of *E. coli* and some pathogen like Salmonella in meat have no conclation. The *E. coli* can acts as indicator for faecal contamination as detected by various tests for *E. coli*, citrobacter, Enterobacter the faecal organism can grow at higher temperature about 44-44.6°C.

2. Direct microscopic examination: The possibility of detecting microbes direct by under microscope shouldn't be missed, helpful in bacterial count/volume, also motility can be detected by having drops, high refractive index of bacterial spores makes them possible to so under phase contrast microscope.

But microbes should be present in large numbers for this, at least 10^6/ml, for milk, yoghurts, fruit juice etc., stained heat fixed smears are prepared and examined for counts of microbes. The advantage of this technique is that it is rapid, although is could not differentiate between living and dead cells.

Recently, DEFT (Direct epifluorescent filter technique) is applied for enumeration of microbes in a variety of foods, although it was originally for milk. Details of it from "examination of milk and milk products."

3.   Application of cultural techniques: Microbes are also examined by encouraging their growth in liquid or surface media. Agar is special substance produced by algae, remains liquid at temperature 40°C, only small amount required to solidity the media (1.5-2%) and lot of advantages.

There are a lot of media available for specific microbes. General purpose media is plate count agars PDA for fungi etc.

Selective media and enrichment media also used. Cooked meat broths incubated at 43°C-45°C allows rapid growth of clustridium perfringens sit becomes dominant.

Some media like Baird-Parkes media are used for isolation of stap¹ ꞈccus aurous. The colony characteristics, biochemical char.   microscopic examinations can be now made and hence, important in food microbiology.

Plate count agar (Aerobic Mesophillic Count), Mc. Conkey broath (for MPN coliform in water), BGLB (Coliforms in food, MPN), Crystal violet-blood agar (For faecal streptococci), Rose Bengal (for moulds and yeasts) etc.

4.   *Enumeration methods:*

(a)   Plate count methods: Do as in milk examination.
(b)   MPN or most probable numbers: based on inoculating replicate tuber of an appropriate liquid medium (3, 4, 5) with three different samples size or dilution of the material to be studied. Then number of the positive tuber are compared with standard charts for probable numbers of bacteria.

A modern variation of MPN is use of hydrophobic grid membrane filter (HGMF), sample is filtered through HGMF into about 1600 small growth compartments or cells after incubation of filter on media, each of cells are counted for growth or number of growth. MPN is applicable to single called organism like bacteria, but not to filamentous fungi because a problem of interpreting the colony forming units separate techniques required for these fungi, e.g. analysis of chemicals like Chetin (compound of cell to all of fungi groups).

5. Alternative methods of examination: The cultural methods are too costly and time consuming, thus food manufactures requires some fast examination techniques for examination of food, some of these are:

(a) *Dye reduction tests*: Same as of milk exhumation.

(b) *Electrical methods*: Activity of Microbes changes chemical and electrical properties of food, electrical properties must frequently monitored are conductance (G), capacitance (C) and impedance (Z). It is possible to take frequent measurements of electrical properties of a medium by growing organism in cell supplied with two metal electrodes. The data can be computer operated and large number of samples can be monitored at same time but large number of bacteria cells (10^6-10^7 cfu/ml) required to initiate a signal. The time taken to reach this number to produce signal (detection time) depends on initial number and growth rate, e.g. *E. coli* incubated at 37°C in Heat infusion broth has detection time of 5-6 hrs. It is a direct test of microbial activity more appropriate then viable count.

(c) *ATP determination*: A number of different living organisms evolved to produce light by activity of Puciferases enzyme of "luciferins" by help of ATP and MgH ions. The reaction produces one photon of light by hydrolysis of one molecule of ATP through a series of intermediates. Now a days such low level emission can be accurately measured. Photomultipliers tubes can detect 10^2-10^3 fg (femtogram) corresponding to 10^2-10^3 bacterial cells.

The results are good with pure cultures but it should be ensured that non-microbial ATP present in food might be separated from detection of microbial ATP. The microbial cells can be removed from liquid food by filtration or centrifugation, but not applied to solid food. Also, there is different amount of ATP in different microbial cell.

So, ATP measurement can not be widely for routine examination of food. There is lot of potential of developing for microbes.

6.   Rapid Method for detection of specific organism and toxins: In the Rapid Method we generally use two method that are immological method and second is DNA/RNA method.

FERMENTED FOOD PRODUCTS

The negative role of microbes is harmful but they also have helpful effects for foods, a number of useful applications in industry, a lot of types of fermented foods used cell over the world. The proper use of modern food technologies and microbiology can produce a good quality of food products with desirable characteristics. It is also helpful for flavour, texture and keeping quality foods. Fermented foods produced in also on small scales as well as industrial scale. The microbes are naturally present in raw food or added as "starters culture". Various chemicals, organic acids like lactic acids etc. produced during fermentation which also process the food.

The lactic acid bacteria are most important applied for fermented milk and dairy products. Yeast are single celled fungi used for fermented products. Some moulds are also participating in production of fermented food products.

(a) *Fermented milk and other dairy products*: There is how-ever, a huge river sity of floods simply that are bees, cheese, *idli*, *sushi*, *kefes*, yoghut, *nam pai*, *duto salami*, *saysavce*, *miso*, *tibi*.

In spite of these mentioned, a lot of other fermented food products like *Busa* (Turkey), *Chicha* (S. America), *Dawadawa* (from *Locust beam*, W. Africa), *Poi* (from Taro, in Hawai), *Puto* (from rice in Philippines) etc. are popular in various part of world.

(b) *Other fermented food products*: A variety of other products also used all over the world. Some important of them are enlisted as below:

1.   *Sauerkraut:* Most of horticultural can be preserve by lactic acid fermentation, e.g. cabbage, cucumbers, oliber, carrots, cauliflower, onion, sweet and hot peppers, green tomato

etc. In Korea fermented vegetables are known as *'kimchi'*. The sauerkraut is produce from lactic acid fermentation of cabbage (*Brassica oleracca*). Under commercial products, lactobacillus cultures are leafy, core and trim, and then shredded 2-5 mm thick. Then it is packed with 2-3% salt in jars or barrels. It is filled into vats, wooden pieces placed one it to keep it submerged (Anaerobic). Action of salts produce causes with draul of juice from vegetables. Thus, it is covered and sealed and allowed ferment and finally pasteurized before packaging. The *Leuconostoc mesenteroides* and *Streptococcus luctis* etc initiate fermentation, produce about 1.0% of lactic acid. Then *Lactobacillus beris* and *L. plantarum* grow and increase acidity up to 2.5%. The acids, esters and diacetyles produced gave pleasant Anema and 21-20°C temperature. The *Pediococcus cerevesiae* also begin to grow rapidly during fermentation.

2. *Pickles:* Preservation of cucumbers and other vegetables as pickles in common practice. It is also a results of lactic acid fermentation from a number of vegetables and fruits. Hence, made pickles uses high salt **ceneem** and vinegar for production. Commercially such raw materials are allowed to ferment lactic acid for preservation. It can be of two types high salt (salt stock) and low salt fermentations stock salt cucumbers are fermented in brine having 5-8% of salt until they are stabilized by conversion of all fermentable sugar into organic acid and other products. The microbes involved are *Lactobacillus brevis*, *L. plantarum* and *Pedococcus pentosaccus*, due to high salts, leucenestoc mesenteroids can not play role as in saurkraut or Kimchi fermentation produced. The fermentation takes about 6-8 week time coleus consistency and flavours of food changes salt stock can be used to prepared are sweet, sour, mixed and other types of pickles.

3. *Fermentation of olives:* These are natives of esteem Mediterranean region. The fruit are treated with brine during which, bitterness is last and fermentation takes place Spanish type grow olives are prep. (38% of worlds production), unsipended fruit treated with lye. They lye

in washed off and kept mesentenoids are previable fermenting organisms.

The traditional grack style product, natural black olives in brine, accounts for 31% of world preservation. The microflora during ripening is dominated by yeasts along with *saccharmyces*. It is undergoing a slow fermenting process lactic acid production is less in comparison to other products.

4. *Idli*: Popular dish in South India prepared from paraboloid rice and decuticled black gram (*Pharcotus mungo*). Ingradients wahsed with H_2O, soaked for some time separately followed by through mixing and grinding. A little salt is added and allowed to ferment for 10-12 hrs. and backed in steam in special containers. Lactic and acetic acid produced along with CO_2. It imparts tasty seur taste to idlys. Predominant microbes involved are *Leuconestoc mesenteriods*, *Streptococcus facralis*, and *Pediococcus cereveriae*.

5. *Ensilage*: It is used for Animals fodder. The finely chopped, partly mature plants like wheats corn or alfa-alfa are packed in tanks or other containers microbes starts growing and fermenting the plant juice carbohydrates firstly, lactis bacteria of enterobacteriaceae predominates. As acidity increases, hemo fermentative acid uric organisms begins to grow. A proteolytic or putrefactive fermentation may occur if high amount of nitrogenous compound in plants. *Clostridium butyricum* can render the ensilage by butyric acids which makes in **rancid**. To awid it plants are mixed with suitable amount of carbohydrates or molasses. Also, cultures of *Lectoborillus* and *Streptococcus lactis* should be added for lactic acid fermentation.

6. *Fermented meats*: Fermented sugar originated from Mediterranean region are also popular in China and South-East Asia. In addition to lactic acid fermentation salting and drying provider specific flavour and also increase shelf-life park, beefs. Mutten are commonly used for purpose curing soils are added to produced cured meats to import colour, taste, tasty, stability and texture of foods, Suasage fermentations ranges from temperature

lactic acid fermentatiton. The nitrate reducing employed are Micrococcus various and staphylococcus carnesus are important.

Microorganism of food: Single are proteins or use of microbial biomass in foods and feeds. Although a number of kinds of microbes are recommended for human consumption, including yeasts, moulds and algae to date only yeasts have been used for food to any extant and then under unusual conditions during II World War, there was shortage of protein and vitamis Germans produced yeasts plants here established in Germany, Switzerland, Finland, Jamaica etc. and it acts as rich source of cheap carbohydrates, proteins and vitamins.

Single Cell Protein (SCP): It is the name given to a variety of microbial products produced by fermentation. The Bacteria, yeasts and algae, produced in massive quantities are attractive source of food for animals and humans. The microbes can be cultivated on industrial wastes or by products as nutrients and yield. Large Cell crop known as single cell protein (SCP). The bacterial cells grow on hydrocarbon wastes from petroleum industry are assure of protein in France, Taiwan, Japan and India. It has been estimated that microbes of yeast produce 25 tonnes of proteins in 24 hr, while 1000 lb steer with synthesize only one lb of protein in 24 hr, and this after consuming 12-20 lbs of plant proteins. Similarly, algae grown in ponds can produce 20 tonnes of protein (dry wt.) per area beam and 20-50 times than corn. The bacteria are usually high in protein contents and have a rapid growth rate. The yeast cell crops harvested from vats used to produce alcoholic beverage have been used to as a food supplement for generation. The attractiveness of SCP as food and feed supplement is because of following factors:

1. Microbes grow very rapidly and produce a high yield, e.g. 100 lbs of yeasts can produce 250 tonnes of protein in 24 hr. and so on.
2. The protein content of microbial cells is very high dried cells are pseudomonas spp. grown on petroleum products have 69% of proteins yeasts cells have a proteins content 40-50% and algae about 20-40%.

3. The protein of related microbes contains all essential amino acids.
4. Some microbes, particularly yeasts have a high vitamin content.
5. The medium for growth of microbes may contains industrial wastes or by produced, e.g. liquid paraffins (hydrocarbon) from oil, refineries spent sulfite liquor from pulp and paper industries, Beat molasses and wood hydrolysates.

But use of microbes as food has some disadvantage also they are as below:

1. Bacterial cells have small size and low density which makes harvesting from fermenting medium difficult industries costly.
2. Bacterial cells have high maleic acid content them yeasts and fungi. This can be detrimental to human beings increasing uric acid level in blood. It may cause uric acid poisoning.
3. It is a general believe that bacteria and other microbes are harmful for human being and animals. An extensive education programme is required to eliminate this misbelief and make pubic interest in this field.

Use of yeast as SCP. Has an advantage of their largest size (early to harvest) over bacterial. Also they have level molic acid contents, high lysine content and have ability to grow at acid pH also to is families from ancient times to produce fermented products. Disadvantages includes level growth rates lower protein contents (45-65%) and lowest methionine content than bacteria.

Use of filamentous fungi. Has advantage of easy harvesting but have limitations in growth rates, lowest protein content and acceptability. Algae has disadvantage having cellulosic cell well not digested by human and also concentrate heavy methods.

The basic contents of SCP are far as, proteins and carbohydrates are ingradients water and other elements like phosphorus and potassium. Also, composition depends upon microbes and substrate employed.

Composition of some representative SCP

Criteria for successful use of SCP:

1. The SCP must be safe to eat.
2. The nutritional value dependent upon amino acid composition should be light.
3. It must be acceptable to general public.
4. It must have the functionality, i.e. characteristics which are found in common staple foods.
5. The economic viability of SCP process is extremely complex and in yet to be demonstrated.

Use of SCP in foods: The inactive dry yeasts (*C. utilis*, and *S. cerevisiae*, *S. uvarum*) are often included in fabricated foods like bakery goods baby foods, soap, meat extenders etc. A part from nutritional value, it imports desirable flavour when added in small count. In active dry yeast preparation are also sold in from of tablets or dry powders.

Use in feeds: The use of yeast as ingredient in feed is also well established. A major portion of buyers yeast produced in USA is used in feeds. A special application is use of active dry yeasts or compressed yeasts in preparation of yeast cultural. The feed supplement is prepared by seeding a cereal grain mash with yeast cells, incubation and drink of fermented milk in such as way that live yeast cells, enzymes and ether sensitive nutritional factors are preserved.

The pet food industries in a major outlet of microbial biomass. The dog feed, cat feed and fish feed is supplemented with yeasts. It will make the product more palatable to the animals.

Manufacture of Dairy Products

Various microbes play an important role in public health and manufacture of different dairy products. They are responsible for many disease, and also important for manufacture of delicious food produced: for this, selected microbes are essential, important milks, butter and cheese.

Fermented Milks: From such earlier times them discovery of micro-organisms, various products like 'butter milk and sour milk' were used in various parts of world for human consumption. The fermented milk was prepared by allowing normal lactic acid producing organism to develop, or by inoculating fresh milk with good quality of fermented milk inoculum. During fermentation, lactic acid produced will 'thickness' or 'curdler' milk and produces desired. However, the nature of product depends upon following factors:

1. The source of milk (i.e. cow, buffalo, goat etc.).
2. The temperature to which milk is heated before inoculation.
3. Kinds of microbes in starter culture.
4. The incubation temperature.

The 1975 per capita consumption of various fermented fluid milks is reported to be 38.5 litre (Haukka, 1976), so constitutes a vital part of human diet, various products are now prepared by technically controlled process, these were known from ancient times. The ancient Sanskrit scriptures of India, vedas describes *'dadhi'* a fermented produced of milk, also existence to seur milk in *Bible*; there is lot of diversity in use of various fermented milk produced in various parts of the world.

Starter lactic cultures for fermented milks: Raw milk have number of microbes, due to uncontrolled activity of microbes, uniformity of products not achieved; so it necessary to carry out controlled fermentation with specific microbes. There specific microbes have been identified. This lead to selection and propagation known cultures, called 'States cultures', for lactic acid fermentation, principle organisms are *streptococcus*, *leuconestoc* and *lactobacillus*.

A starter consists of harmless microbes which upon culturing in milk or milk-based mixer, import desirable and predictable characteristics or flavour and texture attributable to a certain fermented milk product. A single strain culture contains individual stain of bacterial sps. while a mixed/multistrain culture consists of mixture or more then one stam or spp.

Principle Genera of lactic and bacteria: (Other Genera currently include are corynebacterium, Enterococcus, Vagococcus, Tetragenicoccus, Alloiococcus).

Each starter culture over to a specific product. Started must be capable of producing rapidly lactic acid and out growing undesirable contaminates even if single sps. of starter used it is required to used different varieties of same sps. To protect culture from bacteriophages for this lyophilized or other pure culture are stocked by commercial labs are used.

Presently common method of distribution of starts is in from of frozen concentrates: These are frozen at $-196°C$ (liquid N_2) have about 10^{11} organism/ml.

Therapeutic and Health Promoting Activities of Fermented Milk

Consumption of fermented milk is of therapeutic value Metchkenikoff (1908) says that usual coliform and Clostridial bacteria is Gut of man produce putrefactive products which are injurious and cause symptoms of disease. Possibly cause of death at old age. It remedy was to prevent activity of these putrefactors by acidifying intestine with lactic acid. Which might done by fermented milk and introducing *Lactobacillus bulgaricuse* which isolated from Bulgaria fermented milk. But later discovered that *L. bulgaricus* is inferior to *L. acidophilus* in long persistency in guts. The idea of metehkeniko off (Russian) was published in 1908 in book *The Prolongation of Life*.

Sometimes live cultures of lactic acid bacteria are termed as 'Probiotics' for this activity. These also have nutritional value as essential amino acid content of body also increased.

Another beneficial effects ability fermented milk to alleviate condition called 'lactose intolerance'. In infants, in absence of 'lactose' enzymes lactose passes to cover directly and attacked by lactose fermenting microbes producing discomforts flatulence and diarrhoea.

If fermented milk is used these effects are absent or highly reduced. Also yoghurt is observed to cause inhibitory effect on coliform bacteria of body of piglcts and human infants (early recovery from diarrhoea).

Lactic acid bacteria have also been reported to stimulate immune system and various studies have described their ability to active macrophage and lymphocytes, improve level of 1 gA, and production of gamma interferon (mainly by *L. acidophilus*).

It has also been suggested lactic acid bacteria have a hypocholestromic effect and thus reduce possibility of a coronary heat disease.

Atimicrobial Activity of Lactic acid Bacteria (LAB)

They cause inhibitory effect on many microbes thus helps in maintaining healthy food condition in many products. The principle factor responsible are low pH. Production of organic acid bacteriocins, H_2O_2, ethinol nutrient deplecation, and low redox potential. Bacteriocons are bactericidal peptides or protein active against spp. usually close to producing organism, regarded as 'natural preservatives' main bactericin used in nisin by *Lactococcus lactis*. Nisin belogns to a group of antibiotic called 'lantibiotic'.

H_2O_2 is also known for antimicrobial activities its production is not lethal to LAB itself because it is antibiotic fermentation so H_2O_2 is limited by O_2 dissolved in substrate at start of fermentation. In milk H_2O_2 is known to potentiate lactoperoxides antimicrobial system.

Heterofermentic LBS also produced ethanol, through in low concentration have antimicrobial effects.

Also low pH to formation of lactic acid inhibits growth of many microbes. Thus, antimicrobial activities of LABS could not be neglected.

Types of Fermented Milk: They are known by various names in different part of world: may be produced by activity of single of sps. of mixed effected of many sps. So important fermented milk and their properties are described as below:

(A) Cultured butter milk

Strickly, butter milk is a liquid (phospholipid rich) obtained as a by-product during curing of cream. But to obtained a cemistant quality product, it is produced directly by foment of skin or partly skimmed milk. It is acidic refreshing drink with distinct buttery flovours.

The microbes involved are streptococcus lactic or *S. cremoris* with *L⋅⋅⋅lomostoc citrovorum* or *L. dextrencium* (lecomestoc is aroma producing bacteria).

Condition of producing and nature of product: The flowsheet of production given below, Main ingredient are - skim milk, low fat milk, cream condcused skin milk non fat dry milk, culture and slat.

Flowsheet for Manufacture of Butter Milk

During the productions, some medium citrate is also added to improve flavour.

The function of lactic acid *streptococci* is to produce lactic acid giving seur taste and curdling of milk, while Leconastoc provides a volatile and natural products which imports characteristic odour to products, (e.g. acetic acid, acetyl methyl carbinol and di-acetyle) The incubation should be at 22°C, Perfect by the butter milk has characteristic.

Fluidity and the viscosity is directly related to acidity.

Excessive agitation, high temperature storage and contamination results in thinner butter milk.

Defects of Butter Milk

Flat "green", (low acidity and low stem temperature cause); High acid, seur (due high temperature, longer incubation); Lumpiness (due to high acidity, lumpiness). Thick heavy body etc are important defects.

(B) Cultured Sour Cream

The raw material is used is directly the cream. Microbes involved in are same as butter milk, i.e., *streptococci* and *leuconestoes*. Strictly speaking, it is not a fermented milk. But manufacture resembles to that of a cultured milk. The flavour and aroma compounds are also contributed by the starter culture Diagrammatic flow chart of Manufacture is:

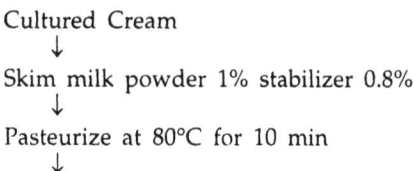

Cultured Cream
↓
Skim milk powder 1% stabilizer 0.8%
↓
Pasteurize at 80°C for 10 min
↓

Hemogenize at 80°C,
 ,↓
13.8 kpa first stage and 3.4 kpa second stage
 ↓
Hot blend seasoning, salt, 80°C
 ↓
Hot pack 75°C seal container
 ↓

Cool to 5°C→Cultured cream clip→Store at 5°C for 3-4 months →seur cream.

(C) Bulgarian Butter Milk

The pasteurized skimmed milk is raw material used. The organism involved is *Lactobacillus bulgarian*.

All inoculated milk is incubated at 37°C rest of all process is same as that of cultured butter milk. The product differs from the commercial butter milk in having higher acidity and lacking Aroma.

(D) Acidophilus Milk

Raw material used is the 'Sterilized Milk'. It requires the organism *Lactobacillus acidophilus* as starter culture. The milk used for propagation of bacteria should be satirized, as it is easily contaminated over by other microbes; the incubation is at 37°C, acidity is allowed to develop to 0.6% - 0.7%.

Whole milk
 ↓
Pasteurize at 90°C for 60 minutes
 ↓
Homogenize at 13.8 kpa
 ↓
Ripening tank = 37°C to pH 4.7
 ↓
Acidophilous milk
 ↓
Bottled
 ↓
Store at 5°C for 3-4 weeks

This milk has therapeutic value, it has ability to trans plant intestinal tract, acidic condition produced by microbes by degradation of lactose will inhibit putrefactive gas producing microbes, microbes is thermophilic hemofomenter but is slow. Firstly VHT given, hold for 3-4 hrs, cooled to 37°C in volume 2-5% added lastly cooled to 5°C for storage. Acidophilous milk is combination with yoghurt is called "Bio-yoghurts" mixed culture used for it, e.g. *L. acidophilous, bifidobacterium,* and *Streptococcus lactus.* So different level acidity and flavour can be produced by mixed combination. Fresh acidophilus milk contain an excess of 500 million cells/ml.

E) Yoghurt/Dahi, Mau, Gioddu

The name 'yoghurt' comes from Turkish word 'Jugurt' which is most available fermented milk in western world today.
Raw material used in milk, skimmed milk or fortified milk to cow, goat, buffalo, sheep etc.

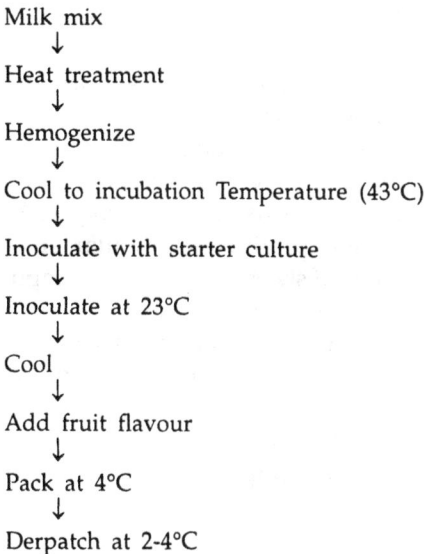

Milk mix
↓
Heat treatment
↓
Hemogenize
↓
Cool to incubation Temperature (43°C)
↓
Inoculate with starter culture
↓
Inoculate at 23°C
↓
Cool
↓
Add fruit flavour
↓
Pack at 4°C
↓
Derpatch at 2-4°C

The microbes involved are streptococcus thermophilous and lactobacillus bulgarious. Remarks - Made from milk in which solids are, concentrated by evaporation of water (some) and addition of skim milk solids; products has consistency resembling custard. Now common in Europe and North America, similar products with different names are produced else where. Milk inoculated with a part of previous batch of yoghurt and heated to 40°-46°C until a thick layer curd develops. Acidity attained 1-3% as lactic acid, all products are non-alcoholic. Detailed study of yoghurt is from percent and Dunn and new food microbiology book.

(F) Kefir

It belongs to a class of product which is partly, acidic fermentation and partly raw material used: Whole milk of cow, goat, buffalo, sheep.

Microorganism involved = *Streptococcus lactis*, lactobacillus, bulgaricus, *L. brevis*, and lactose fermenting yeasts (e.g. *Saccharomyces delbruecei*).

Comments and Remarks: It is mixed lactic acid and alcoholic fomentation bacteria produce 0.6-1% lactic acid and yeasts produce 0.5-1% of alcohol. The organism conglomerate to from granules called 'Kefir grains'. In Balkans, fermentation is carried out in leather bags made of goat skin at a temperature of 25°C, grain can be dried and stored for longer periods.

Kefir is popular in USSR (former), the microbes are added as 'Kefir grains' which are white to yellow coloured, insoluble in H_2O. There are in fact sheets compared of strong polysaccharide 'Kefiran' which folds on itself producing globular structure resembling cauliflower, out side of sheets is smooth and populated by *lactobacillus*, while inner rough side has yeasts and lactic acid bacteria. Many yeasts like Candida kefir, Saccharomyces cereneae and S. exiguus are associated, milk is homogenized and heated to 85-95% for 2-10 minutes, cooled to 22°C, kefir grains added, up to 5%, fermentation for 8-12 hours. In addition to lactic acid, ethanol also presents as flavour components.

(G) Koumiss

It is also acid and alcoholic fermentation products.

Raw Material   = Mare's milk is used.

Microorganism   = Same as in kefir.
Comments   = Product famous in Russia.

Koumiss is fuzzy greyish white milk. It has acidity up to 1.4% and ethanol up to 2.5%. A mixed yeast/Lab flora used. Mare's milk is low in cream concert and don't curdles like cow's milk; starter comists of *lactobacillus* bulgarious and lactose fermenting yeasts. Torulopsis holmi, sometimes horse flesh or some vegetable matter is also added to impart specific flavour. Now- a-days skimmed cows milk used for koumiss production.

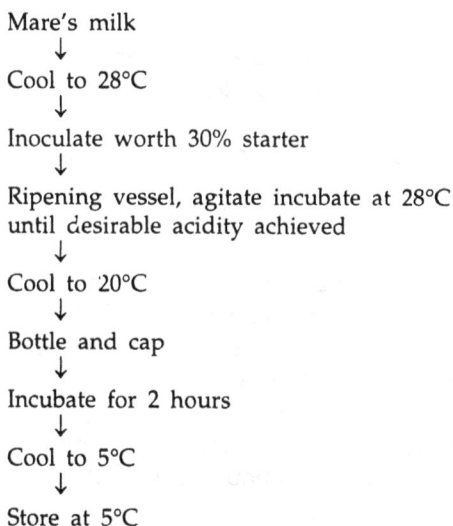

Mare's milk
↓
Cool to 28°C
↓
Inoculate worth 30% starter
↓
Ripening vessel, agitate incubate at 28°C
until desirable acidity achieved
↓
Cool to 20°C
↓
Bottle and cap
↓
Incubate for 2 hours
↓
Cool to 5°C
↓
Store at 5°C

(H) Laben

Whole milk of cow, goat, sheep and buffalo is used. The microbes are same as above. The laben is popular in Egypt.

Manufacture of Butter as important Milk Product

Made by churning pasteurized sweet or sour cream, main principle is to separate out fat globules from other constituents. The liquid portion, butter milk is drained off and granules are further processed. Butter consists of about 80% fats, small percentage of lactose and proteins, and often 2% salt. Remaining is water in the form of minute droplets dispersed through out the butter fat, is dissolved in this water.

The yield of butter as follows: The cream from which the butter is extracted as churned and may be soured naturally by addition of starter for characteristic Arpma, flavours and better yield. Before a starter is added, cream is pasteurized at 71°C for 30 minutes. This eliminates undesirable microbes and destroys milk lipase that would other wise cause rancidity during storage of butter. The starter culture consists of two type of organisms:-

1. These responsible for acidity i.e. *Streptococcus lactis* and *S. cremons.*
2. These imparting characteristics Aroma and flavour, e.g. *Leuconestoc citjonicum* and *L. dextranicum.*

Once pH reaches to 4.3 due to production of lactic acid, Leuconestoc stater causing its growths but its enzymes attacks the citrals and change them into diacetyl compounds. Develop of characteristic Aroma and flavour.

The keeping quality of butter is good. Although it had retained bacteria in cream it is low in sugar and protein. Salted butter, due to high percentage of salt will presents microbial spoilage of butter in compound to in salted butter. Today butter is made from pasteurized cream due to which most of spoilage microbes is destroyed. Also butter is kept refrigerated and during commercial scale storage it is kept about −17.8°C, therefore no microbial growth.

Also water droplets are so eventually distributed and minute that bacteria present in these droplets can't multiply because of space limitations. Another factor which resists microbial growth in presence of anaerobic conditions except the surface.

Undesirable Changes in Butter

Sometimes produced for example

(A) Flavour defects

Mainly came from cream which may receive such flavours from feed of cows, absorb from atmosphere or develop them from incubation. Feeds like onions, french weed, pepper grass etc. congae off flovours, growth of microbes in cream may produce.

(i) Cheesiness caused by *factobacilli*.
(ii) Rancidity resulting from fat splitting bacteria (Lipulysis) by lipase enzyme.
(iii) Barny flavour, produced by Acrobacter sps.
(iv) Multy flavour, produced by *steptococcus lactis*, var-maltigens.
(v) Multy flavour, produced by moulds and Actinomycetes.
(vi) Flat flavour resulting from destruction of di-acetyl by bacteria like pseudomonas etc. The butter may directly have 'surf and tints' or 'rabbito' caused by pseudomonas, introduced by wash water or churning equipments.

Fishiners' in butter caused by *P. iclathyesmia*, 'skunlike flavours' caused by *P. mephitica*. Roquefort like flavour due to moulds.

Rancidity is produced by lipase. Fishiners due to production of trimethylamine from lecithin tallowiners from oxidation of fat catalyzed by bacterial enzymes.

(B) Colour Defects

Pink colour caused by action of SO_2 refrigerant; surface darkening from loss of water from surface. Surface discolouration result by activity of bacteria, yeast or moulds specially in unpasteurized cream.

Dark smoky and greenish areas when *Alternaria* or Claderporium grows, brown areas by phoma or *Alternaria*; fusarium culmorum causes bright, reddish pink grease, etc.

The microbes spoilage butter can be grouped as:

1. *Yeast and Moulds*: e.g. Yeast is gerera Torula, and moulds like *Asporigillus, Mucor, Rhizopus, Cladosperium* and *Altermaria*.
2. *Proteolytic organism*: Many spese fermers like Micrococci cause destruction of casein and produce undesirable changes.

3. *Lipolytic organisums:* Like Pseudomonas, Alcaligenes, serratia, Micrococcus, Achromabacter are lipolytic, fact is hydrolysed and a pungent odour and flavour develops.
4. *Coliform organism:* Presence of Enterobacter anageneses and *E. coli* indicates pest pasteurization contamination. They produce acid and gas.

Microbial examination of butter is limited yeast and moulds are objectionable samples with less then 10 yeast/moulds per gram are solid to be good. The number of proteolytic bacteria should be less than 50/g.

The examination is done by use of specific media for different microbes, and plate, count is done accordingly.

Manufacture of Cheese as Fermented Dairy Product

Cheese can be defined as consolidated curd of milk fat is entrapped by coagulated easein. Unlike fermented milk, physical characteristic of cheese are for removed from these of milk, because protein coagulation proceeds to a greater extent due to proteolytic enzymes. Cheese is basically means of storing milk and has been used from along time. A detailed idea of cheese making and a variety of cheese given by Mair-woldbrug (1974A) and Walter and Hatgove (1969).

Historical development of cheese and its origin was undertaken. It is speculated that ancient man has slaughtered product because after sucking milk of its mother by action of remain. Also, there are evidences that man domesticated shop around 9000 years before Christ in Iran.

Cheese is actually the product made by separation of casein from the liquid. It is a valuable means of conserving nutrients in the milk. Brilent-Savarin (1755-1826) that "Dissert without cheese is like a pretty woman with only one eye". It reveals importance of cheese. Today cheese making is a major industry cell over world, producing about 10 million tonnes per annum. Among various types of cheese, chedden cheese is commercially most important and produced on large scale all over would due to its qualities.

Manufacture of Cheese

Manufacture depends upon activity of selected microbes. Different varieties are manufactured by providing suitable conditions and/or these microbes. The quality of cheese is determined by biochemical activities of these microbes. The quality of cheese is determined by biochemical activities of these microbes.

Milk Used For Production of Cheese

Whole milk of skimmed milk (mostly of court) used, rapidly delivered to production sites; it should be free from antibiotic residues, other chemical contaminations are serious off Flavours, also should bot have excessive growth of psychrophilic microbes. It necessary heat treatment is given to the milk to ensure safe products, also given in "Standard Methods of Examination of Dairy Products".

Starter Culture and Inoculation

Milk is added with starter cultures, having one or more spp. of lactic acid bacteria, the acid produced by these in early stages facilities clotting of milky coagulant. Mostly are mesophilic startes e.g. Stages of *Lactobacillus laetis* or *Streptococcus cremoris* if mesophilic conditions (below 38°C). Themophlic startes as *Lactobacillus helveticus*, *L. casei*, *L. delbrueekek*. *L. bulgarieus*, and *streptococcus salvarius* for production at higher temperatures (up to 50°C) e.g. for Swiss cheese role of starter culture is crucial and complex; major function is to convert lactose to *lactic acid*, decrease in pH, produce sharp flavour, stability of colloidal suspension of casein is weakened and calcium released from casein miecller.

Forming calcium lactate also, some other microbes like propioni bacterium shermani for swiss cheese and moulds for blue or camembert cheese. They have important function during ripening process: Mostly good quality frozen culture are suitable for cheese production.

Use of Coagulant

A coagulant is added to milk after 30 minutes addition of starter culture. It is an enzyme that splits colloidal casein into a carbohydrate-rich peptide fraction and the insoluble paracasein that precipitates in presence of Cr^{++}.

Mostly, rennet extract (Renin) obtained from calves stomach is used, also called casein coagulase, alternative coagulants used due to shortage of calves blench of e.g. cow and coagulants of fungal origin have now been used.

Cutting of Coagulum

Rectangular formes with thin wires used for cutting the coagulum into microbes. Thus, tacilitering less of 'whey' which is also new easy to heat and process further the cheese.

After coagulation, watery fluid separates out having 93%, H_2O, 5% lactose + small amount of other dissolved granules. It is called 'whey' and is a by product. It can be used after dehydration therefore only lactose and granules remained.

(i)   Can be used as a fodder supplement for domestic animals, sold in powder form.
(ii) Also used in lactic acid and other fermentation processes.

Cooking of Cut Coagulum

Cubes in curd suspended in 'whey' heated to origin temperature for a specific time (37-38°) to 30 minute for cheddar cheese stiring is also done, Thus cubes contracts and express free whey. Cooking also controls acid acid production by starter culture, and suppress growth of spoilage bacteria.

Draining of 'Whey'

A complished whey by draining whey from vat that contain whey-curd mix, precaution taken to present less of curd. During man time of removed. Some lactic acid is produced by starter cultures. The curd may remain in Vat. So some knitting of curd particles can occur as in case of cheddar cheese. During kintting, curd particles clearly adhere to each other having a fine texture.

Salting of Curds

Salting (NaCl) is done one or several ways. Dry salts may be sprinkled on loose curds. (Casein cheddar) or fresh cheese can be immersed in proper aqueous solution of salt, or rubbing on surface of pressed cheese, salting provides following importance.

1. In genes flavours and taste.
2. Controls moisture and appearance of other.
3. Presents undesirable microbes.
4. Controls moisture content withdraw of H_2O.
5. Control production of lactic acid.

Pressing of Curd

It may be before of afterward of salting for this, hydrophilic pressure of weights can be used P. ling of cheese in Vat (*cheddan*) is a kind of hydrolic pressure.

Pressing haves cheese a characteristic shape and compactness. Vacuum chambers can be used to remove occulated air from cheese and gave production closely knit body.

Ripening of Cheese

Finished cheese is allowed for ripening to develop characteristic aroma and flavour. During this, composition and physical properties-changes due to microbes and their enzyme. The nature of changes depends upon microbes or present temperature and relative humidity of curing rooms. Various microflora are developed during ripening depending upon type of flavour required.

During ripening degradation of lactose, proteins and fats takes place by microbes. Lactose is changed into lactic acid + alcohol + volatile acids + natural products. In soft cheese, protein is completely degraded into peptides and amino acids. This lipases elaborated by moulds hydrolyses fats releasing biotitic, caprylic capric, capric and higher fatty acid. So, causes development of desired flavours, Aroma and texture.

Now, cheese can be packed and preserved at low temperatures before marketing.

Now, *Nature of Cheese*: Depends on moisture content. If 'Whey' is 'Separated out' from perforated moulds, curd would-be 'soft' because it is only 'drained off'. It has high moisture contents. The low moisture cheese preparation by heating, pressurizing and cutting of pieces hard cheese is prepared.

Type of Cheese Sold in Market

Depending upon the moisture fact contents, condition of storage and types of micro-organism required.

- (A) Soft cheese or cottage type or cream cheese: There is no ripening, used freshly prepared. If we add cream during curdling. It is called cream cheese.
- (B) Hard/Dipend/Rennet Curd cheese: It has low moisture content. It is ripened by enzyme and slow growth of bacteria or moulds or both.
- (C) Semisoft cheese or it is ripened by proteolytic and/or lipolytic microbes which soften the curd and gene it flavours.

(A) *Soft or Cottage Type Cheese*: The majority types are:

(1) Cottage types or soft acid curd type.
(2) Cream cheese.

The manufacture of this cheese is almost similar to that of General method. Prepared from pasteurized skim milk or skim milk powder. The pasteurization is at 72°C for 15 seconds. New small amount (5%) of starter culture and then some little rennet or coagulator added in Vat. After curdling, curd is cut into cubes using wire knives. The whey is drained 'off' and cottage cheese is prepared. Curd is cooked, washed and mixed with salt and cream dressing.

Moisture should be less than 80%, and milk fats should be at least 4%. Some silicones sortrate etc. preservaties used.

This starter culture includes mix of *Leucomestoc citrovorum* and *L. dextranicum* (for flavour and aroma) and *streptococcus lacits* for lactic acid. Heating is done at 50°C and then H_2O is added that, curd settler down during manufacture.

(A) *Cream Cheese*: Cream cheese has at least 33% milk fats and maximum of 55% moisture. Ingradients used are cream, milk skim milk, condensed milk prepared by cooked curd process similar to cottage cheese. Its derivation is due to growth of yeast and moulds.

(B) *Hard or Ripened or Rennet Curd Cheese*: It is properly ripened by moulds and bacteria. It may be American cheddar type, Edam cheese or swiss cheese.

(i) American cheddar type cheese: It is also known as 'yellow cheese' by addition of edible colours made in cylindrical and block shapes filling curd into steel barrels. The slight differences in process of its manufacturing are:

(a) After slight acidity develops due to starter *S. cremoris* and *S. lacttis*, renned is added. This makes the cheese 'elastic'. Now curd becomes firmed. The 'whey' is drained off and used for stock feed. The 'clumps' or masser of cheese are chopped again and piledup. This 'chopping' and 'piling' is known as 'cheddaring'.

Now salting is done, and it is pressed into heops for ripening at storage roomes (2-15°C, 85%, relative humidity). Now, sharpening is done with a knife (of edges).

Ripening is done depending upon organism we use. Generally proteolytic and lipolytic organism used. Products of these bacteria gene characteristic odour and flavour, e.g. Diacetyl, lactic acid, butyric acid, caproic acids. Acetic acids and various amines.

Many of them also produce vitamins, like Nicotinic acid, vitamin B-Complex etc. increasing the nutritive value of cheese. Various bacteria like *Lactobacilli lacits*, *L. acidophlius*, *L. pentosus*, *Micrococcus frendenreichei*, *streptococcus liquifaciens*, and *S. durans* etc. also add to flavour of cheddar cheese.

If there are defects in manufacture gases will be produced due to contamination with clestridium, *E. coli* etc.: undesirable off flavour produced and is called as 'Gray cheese'.

(b) *Swiss Cheese/Emmentales Cheese*: It undergoes double from fermentation: The lactic acid and propionic acid fermentation. Production of some gas is essential for development of 'eye' of cheese.

The starter cultures used are Thermoduric bacteria a like *streptococcus lactis, lactobacillus vulvarious, Propioni bacterium* shermanii, *pseudomonas fruedenrcichii* etc. after cutting curd cheese into pieces, it is cooked to 50°C, salting done by soaking cheese in brine solution of 23°C salts, for some days at 13°C.

Ripening is done by spp. of propionibacterium when incubated at 22°C for few months. Due to this 'eye' develops as a result of CO_2 formed by activity of propioni bacterium. This cheese has flavour is a bitter sweet taste. The typical flavour is caused by formation of glycerol and propionic acid and succinic acids.

(c) *Semisoft Cheese*

    (a)   Requestor cheese/Gorgenzola cheese/blue cheese (Mould Ripened)
    (b)   Comembert cheese
    (c)   Limburges cheese
    (d)   Liederkarnz cheese.

Requefort or bule cheese or soft ripened cheese It contains high fat and slat contents for preservation from contamination. Salt content is up to 5%. It is ripened by species of mould Penicillium roqueforti. It is introduced in from of inoculum of spores. The fungus grows inside cheese forming blue green conidia and sharp flavour develops. The sps of mould is aerobic. Thus preformation made in cheese when it is spread out on hoops itself.

For other 3 varieties, ripening is done by growth of microbes in form of red orange slimy coatings on outer surface. In case of Limburgen when acidity is produced by lactic acid. This yeast begin to grow for about a week, It is surface ripened variety of cheese.

General Type of Industrial Processes

There are various types of industrial processes where microorganism are used to produce desirable and products. Which have well defined industrial uses and applications. These many uses be broadly dressified into the following groups:

(1) Foods and Food Additives

Micro-organisms themselves are cultivated on a large scale for use as food and the animal feed. Most fungi and algae are produced from media containing nitrogenous source and other readily available and cheap nutrients. Such food producer are good sources of protein, vitamins, and other organic nutrients. In recent years microbial processes are employed for range scale production of amino acids.

(2) Alcoholic Beverages

Fruit juices and extract of grains are fermented with the production and beer, wine and other alcoholic beverages.

(3) Manufacture of Various Chemicals

Microorganisms ferment various substances, usually carbohydrates, in nutrient media. They produce a variety of chemicals (various alcohols, lactic acid, acetic acid, citric acid, gluconic acid etc.) which are being recovered, purified and solution.

(4) Therapeutic Compounds

Antibiotic, vitamins and steroidal drugs are prominent this category.

(5) Industrial Compounds (Enzymes)

A number of microbial enzyme have industrial applications and are produced on a large scale.

In addition to these, there are other processes converted with micro-organisms, or where micro-organism are used for special industrial purpose. The principles and practices of these processes are comparable in may ways to those of industrial microbiology. For example deterioration of textiles, leather, metal, plastic, rubber, wood and wood products is a manor concern of industry. However, micro-organisms are used in processes. Such as retting and flax, preparing hides for leather and coffee bean-hulling.

Another aspect of industrial microbiology is large scale cultivation of pathogenic micro-organisms for the preparation of vaccines through this is not a fermentation process. Analytical microbiology is another field of industrial microbiology where micro-organism are used for quantitative analysis of antibiotics, vitamins and amino acids.

Food and Food Additives Beaker's Yeast

The production of beakers yeast is the biggest domestic use of a micro-organisms for food purpose. Beakers yeast is a stram of saccaromyces cerevisease. The strain of yeast in carefully selected for its capacity and produce eggs quickly, its liability during ordinary storage, and its ability and produce desirable flavour. The organisms are mixed with bread dough is being about vigorous sugar fermentation is responsible for leaving bringing the dough.

A pure culture of selected strain of yeast is first grown in the laboratory gradually built up to large and large volume of transfer from the test tube to the fermentor tank. Great care is taken is prevent contamination at any stage of development of culture. During manufacturing, the stain is inoculated into a medium which frequently contains molasses and cornsteep liquor as source of carbon, nitrogen and minerals salts. The reaction of the medium is adjusted to pH 4.4 to 4.6. The incubated medium is incubated at a temperature of 25-26°C, and is aerated during the incubation period. Yeasts oxidize sugars under aerobic conditions with the liberation of energy. A large part of this is utilized for the synthesis of cell protoplasm. The yeast cells multiply rapidly and exhaust the sugar supply within 10 hrs.

At the and of incubation yeasts cells are removed from the fermented medium by centrifugation, washed and mixed with starch or corn meal, and them being pressed into cake from. Yeast cakes must be kept cool is preserve the cells and is prevent spoilage by other micro-organisms. They may also be dried. Dried yeast remains viable for several months. Yeast are rich in vitamins and most of the essential amino acids required by man and animals.

Food and Fodder Yeast

Yeast propagated essentially for food purpose is known as food-yeast. Yeast produced chiefly and feed animals is called fodder-yeast. The mass cultivation of yeast for use as food, more specifically as a food supplement is to compensate for the dietary inadequacies in the regions of the world where human molnution is chronic. Secondly, there is great emphasis and interest on lowering the BOD of the effluents from industrial plants. Thus, several processes to manufacture yeast from industrial and agricultural wastes have been undertaken. This con wastes time prevents environmental pollution.

Single Cell Protein (SCP)

SCP is the name given to a variety of microbial products that are produced by fermentation. When properly produced, this material makes satisfactory proteinaceous ingradients for animal food or human, food. The most recent micro-biological industry. Yeasts, fungi, bacterial and algae are grow on hydrocabon wastes, and cells are harvested as source of protein. It has been calculated that 100 hrs of yeast will produce 250 tonnes of proteins in 24 hours.

(1) Bacterial cells have smaller size and low density, which makes harvesting from the fermented medium difficult and costly.

(2) Bacterial cells have nuclic acid content relative is yeast and fungi. Thus, can be detrimental to human beings lending to increase. The uric acid level in blood. This may lead uric acid poisoning or gout. To decrease the nuclic acid level additional Processing step has to be introduced, and this makes it costly.

(3) The general public thinking is that all bacteria are harmful and produce diseases. An extensive education programme.

Milk Microbiology

Milk and its composition: Milk is the normal secretions of mammary glands of mammals excluding colostrum. It is mainly meant for the nourishment of their young children. It is almost a complete food: and also an excellent medium for growth of many micro-organisms.

The colostrum (first milk) is much more concentrated fluid containing up to 25% of total solids, many proteins, secreted immediately after parturition. A number of animals are used for human consumption of milk, but cows and buffaloes are most prominent.

The principal components milk are water, proteins, fat and lactose. However, freshly drawn milk from cattle varies in their composition. This variation is due to following reasons:

1. Species of mammal,
2. Breed of mammal,
3. Age of individual,
4. Stage of location,
5. Feed of animals,
6. Year's reason.

And also the health of animal.
The average composition of milk is given as below:

Water	87.3%
Lactose	5%
Butter fat	3.8%
Casein	2.5%
Albumin and globulin	0.7%
Mineral (ash)	0.7%
pH	6.7 to 6.9
Specific gravity	1.035

Generally, protein content of milk reflect the growth rate of animal, *i.e.*, higher the growth rate, the more protein milk contains.

Besides this composition, milk also contains vitamin A, B, (Thiamene) and B_2 (riboflavin). It also contains trace of vitamin 'C' and 'D'. Hence, provides an excellent medium for many bacterial species.

Usually, sterile skimmed milk (fat fra) is used for growth and maintenance of microbes on lab.

Table 2.1given below shows the composition of typical milk.

Typical Milk Composition [% weight/l]

A detailed analysis of 'cow's milk reveals that lipid content is most variable. About 80-85% of milk protein is in the from of casei. These are five main classes of casein (α_{s1}, α_{s1}, β, r, k) which aggregates together in addition of calcium phosphate in milk to from colloidal portion known as micelles. Balance of protein made up of whey proteins which mainly comprise the globular proteins β lactoglobulin and α lactalbumin and also a number of blood deried proteins.

Table 2.1
Composition of Typical Milk

Fat	Protein	Lactose	Total	Solids
Human	3.8	1.0	7.0	12.4
Cow	3.7	3.4	4.8	12.7
Jerry	5.1	3.8	5.0	14.5
Ayrrhire	4.0	3.5	4.8	13.0
Short hern.	3.6	4.9	4.9	12.6
Sheep	7.4	5.5	4.8	19.3
Goat	4.5	2.9	4.1	13.2
Water buffalo	7.4	3.8	4.8	17.2
Horse	1.9	2.5	6.2	11.2

Cattle's Milk

It is always sterile when it is drawn but it gets contaminated the time when it is dispensed into containers for commercial purposes, for contamination, the healthy cattle's milk should be sterile, but if contaminated with a number of microbes at the time of hardling and processing, various microbes in milk will degrade milk components like fats, proteins or carbohydrates. Hence, the product becomes unpalatable, (the taste becomes seur and also unpleasant oil our may be present). If contaminated by microbes, becomes unfit for consumption, and may be responsible for a number of milk, borne epidemics, e.g. Typhoid lever, Diphtheria, TB, poliomyelitis, foot and mouth disease, Brucellosis salmonellosis, etc., but apart from there microbes some microbes also brings about desirable changes in milk to produce various products like butter, cheese, curd yogurt etc. Thus it is quite important to study about microflora of milk for public health and commercial purpose.

Importance of Study of Milk Microbiology

These are few important points of significance of studying milk microflora:

1. To judge sanitary quality and conditions of milk and milk products.
2. Micro-organisms of milk, under suitable conditions, degrade milk components like proteins, fats and carbohydrates, making milk unpalatable.
3. Many milk born epidermic caused by milk micro-organisms.
4. Some microbes produce desirable changes resulting in production of butter, cheese, etc. some desirable effects of milk microbes are "blue milk" (pseudomonas cyenogenes). 'Red milk' (Serratia marcensecesns) or 'ropiness' (Alcaligenes viscosus) or sometimes milk appears duity or stale, sometimes 'off' flavours also develops in milk.

Sources of Micro-Organisms of Milk

When milk is drawn out from cattle - it still contains a number of microbes like bacteria etc., which entered into teat canal. That's way some milk is discarded out initially. These bacteria are mechanically 'flushed out' during milking. Right from the time milk is drowned, until dispeured into containers and manufacture of various products, there are number of factors which come in contact are sources of milk contamination, certain strict hygienic conditions can reduce the population of milk microbes.

In fact, milk does possesses a number of antimicrobial features either to protect the udder from infection or to protect new born calf, Generally, there are present at too law a concentration in milk to have a very market effect on its keeping quality or safety. In some cases, antimicrobial activity is antagonized by either milk constituents such as effect of citrate and bicarbonate on lactoferrin activity. Some important sources of milk contamination are:

(A) The Producing Animal

Many times, animal is itself responsible for contamination. Thus health of producing animal is of prime importance. Unless like flanks, udder and teats are specially cared, there are much chances of milk contamination, some bacteria comes on teat opening and may enters easily the "under interior". Aseptically drawned cow's milk contains low number of organisms, fevoer than 10^2-20^3 cfu/ml. The common microbes are micrococci, streptococci, and coryebacterium bevies. The bacterial count increase if animal is infected by disease of udder called "Mastitis". It is major cause of economic less in dairy industry, about, 90 million annually in England and Wales. The bacterial count may rise up to 10 cfu/ml. Mastitis is also diagnosed by rise of polymorphonuclear leukocyted which may be 10^7/ml in infected milk. This inflammatory disease of under may also contributes to blood cells in milk. If cattle is suffering from disease, milk should not be consumed but is must be drawn out of cattle or otherwise, it may spoil out in udder and damagcit due to increased bacterial counts.

Important microbes causing Mastitis are *Staphylococcus aureus, E. coli, Streptococcus agulactiae, Pseudomonas acruginosa* etc.

Thus, washing and massage of udder with warm, detergent sanitizer solution is important to prevent disease.
The Hair, dust and dirt of animals also has bours a number of microbes. These may be unknowingly added to the milk in the equipments also like 'pails' (or buckets), milking machines, milking cupts etc.

If such microbes are pathogenic, they may become cause of epidemics. Thus, periodic examination of milk is very essential.

(B) Milking area as a Source of Microbes: i.e., exterior of udder and surrounding area

The microbial content of milking contamination; by many practices like feeding operation etc. The problem is intensified when allowed to graze in open pastured or kept indoor wet conditions, heavily infected terts contributes 10^5 cfu/ml. Increased momentary activities raise dust in air, increasing chance of contamination. Thus, environment should be kept clean and hygienic. The contamination fem bedding and manure can be source human pathogen like *E. coli*, camplobacter, salmonella etc.

These should be proper monitoring, of bacterial count of air time to time and accordingly, precautions must be taken.

(C) Milk Handling Equipments and Utensils:

Unhygienic equipments and utensils are known to be most important source of milk contamination. The teat cups, pipe works, milk holders and storage tanks are principal source of milk contamination. Specially, interior of such equipments are primary source of contamination. They may be accounts to lakhs to billions of microbes/ml of milk. It not properly cleaned, they acts as primary source of contamination. Milk is a nutritious medium and if not properly cleaned these equipments nourish the microbes on surfaces and also contaminations fresh batches of milk. So proper somatization and treatments should be applied. If cleaning is neglected for long times, the hydrophilic, mineral rich deposit called "Milk stone' develops on surface of interior. They are 'sanitizes proof' and allows growing micrococci and enterococci to develop.

The containers having crackles, crevices, dents are among major habitat of microbes along with scratches and other irregularities.

Thus, suitable washing methods for the equipments should be applied, e:g. warm water and sanitizer solution with help of a branch.

For milking machines, other methods applied, e.g. stream or hot water treatment, or passage of chloride or quaternary.

Ammonium Compen Like Dilute Casly Solution:

(D) Personnel Source of Contamination

The persons involved in the milking area should be healthy and aware of personnel hygienic. Before drawing, hands should be properly washed, cleaned and rinsed in bactericidal solution, dry them with-clean, Towel. The fingers nails should cutted and dust free before any practice, a neat and clean uniform, and have a handkerchief to present direct conghing a sneezing. Use of a surgical masle as an additional measure. Personnel contamination is not much, but may lead to addition of human pathogens and cause epidemics. The persons infected from diseases or carriers etc. are sources. The importance of personal hygiene is to prevent harmful microbes in milk and spread as epidemics.

(E) Water as Sources of Contamination

Water is continuously used for various purposes in dairy industry. So special attention should be given for clean water supply at dairies etc. Water is used for cleaning untensils, washing of hands and also feeding of cattle. Thus, water quality should be maintained which is decided by source of supply. The surface H_2O is always contaminated with dust plants and debris of dead animals etc. Thus, quality of water should be continuously monitored.

Test For Water Quality

The test used is "presumptive coliform Test" to check potability. The coliform group of bacteria like *E. coil* may present for this chlorination of water is commonly practised to are potability.

The Milk Marketing Board (MMB) of England and Wales introduced a system of payment to dairy owners based on TBC (Total Bacterial Count) various categories of milk are divided and at present 76% of milk there is of category 'Bond A' which means count 1.7×10^3 cfu/ml.

In developed countries, milk after drawing is immediately chilled before transporting it for further processing.

Types of Micro-organism in Milk

A number of microbes are present in the milk, depending on specific conditions and batch of milk, *e.g.* Bacteria, Fungi. Moulds, Yeasts, bacteriophage and even protozoans but protozoans are seldom observed. There microflora of milk are described as below:

(A) Bacteria

Most common, e.g. cocci (usually gram+ve), Gram+ve non-spore forming rods, and Gram+ve spore forming rods as well as gram+ve non-spore forming rods. There are many examples: *Streptococcus lactis, Enterococci, Pseudomonas aeurginosa* and other sp., Salmonella, Micrococcus, clostridium, corynebacterium pyogens etc. The pathogenic bacteria like mycobacterium bevies and mycobacterium tuberculosis may also be present.

(B) Yeast

Most frequently encountered in milk. They acts upon lactose and produces lacitc acid and carbon dioxide, e.g. Torula species, most commonly found on raw cream in hot weather, but prevails through out the year also.

(C) Molds

Grows in large concentration and appears as fluffy or fuzzy growth; sometimes appears on surface of milk product like butter, cream, *khoa* or cheese etc. produce undesirable flavours and odours, but certain moulds are essential for production of typical type of cheese.

(D) Bacteriophages

These are particularly obnoxious (*i.e.,* harmful) and can be seen in starter cultures of cultured milk, butter and cheese, they kills bacterial cultures and process or formation of fermentation product nil stops.

Classification of Milk Microflora or Physio-Chemical Pasis

(A) On Basis of Bio-Chemical Activities

Microbes are able to bring about various biochemical change in raw milk, they may be lipolytic proteolytic or acid producers etc. During normal fermentation, a characteristic and sour flavours develop in milk by *Streptococcus lactis* and *S. cremosis* by conversion of lactose to lactic acid.

The bacteria producing only one type of acid are Hemofermentive e.g. lactic acid is the major fermentation product due to *S. lactis* and *S. cremosis* and certain *lactobacill,* the microbacterium, coliforms also ferments lactose to lactic acid and other products.

Hetero fermentive organisms. They produces acid propionic acid. Acetic acid gases like H_2CO_2 alcohol etc. Lactic acid continues to form until to be comes limiting factor for bacteria itself. As acidic reaches 4.7 pH precipitation of casein takes place eand organism able to metabolize lactic acid develops spirally acid one yeast and moulds, acidity diminished, alkaline product of protein decomposition like amines, ammonia product e.g. by species of bacillus, clostridium, pseudomonas etc.

Sometimes, changes non-deleterious to health are also bring about by microbes, e.g. Ropiness or slimness (to be polled into threads) by 'Alcahgenes viscolactis' a 'tapid' or 'stormy' fermentation of lactose by clostridium perfringous some organisms imparts brilliant colours to milk, e.g. pseudomonas syscyanea (blue) pseudomonas synxantha (yellow) and seriatia marcerceris (red colour).

Biochemical Types of Organism in Milk

They may be classified into five major types.

Type I Acid Producers: The representative microbes are:

(1) Septococci like streptococcus lactic acid and S cremosis.

- Source or these microbes are Dairy utemils. Manure equipments udder etc.
- The activity (biochemical) involves easily scuring of milk, conversion of lactose to lactic acid and other products, may be homo or hetero fermentive, produces also the acetic acid, propionic acid etc. and alcohol with CO_2.

(2) Lactobacilli

(i) Example: *Lactobacillus casi, L. Planterum, L. brevis, L. fermentum.*
(ii) Source: feeds, silage and manure.

(iii) Bicochemical activity: Lactose fermented to 2-1% lactic acid, some are homo and other are heterofermentive.

(3) *Microbacterium*

(i) Example: *Microbacterium lacticum.*
(ii) Source: Manure dirty utensils dairy products.
(iii) Activity: Produce lactic acid and other product. lactic acid is less produced as composed to steprococci or lactobacilli, some of microbacteria can survive even at temperature 80-85°C for 10 minutes.

(4) *Coliform Group*

(i) Example: *Escherichia coli, Enterobacter aerogones* etc.
(ii) Source: Manure, polluted water soil and plants.
(iii) Activity: They are heterifermentire, *i.e.* other products like gases, alcohols etc. are also produced along with lactic acid neutral product also produced and number of coliform bacteria milk is indicator if its sanitary quality.

(B) *Biochemical Type II Gas Producers*

(1) Coliforms like *Clastridrum butysicum* and *Torula ceremoris*:

(a) *Source*: Soil, manure, water and feed
(b) *Activity*: Lacture fermented with accumulation of gas, gas may be a mixture of $(CO_2 + H_2)$ or only CO_2 in case of yeast fermentation.

The bulk containers of milk may here their lids lifted by gas pressure when contamination is high.

(C) *Bicochemical Type-II*

Repy or stringy fermentation

(a) *Examples*: *Alcaligenes viscolactis, Enterotractes aerogenes, Steptococcus cremoris* etc.

(b) *Sources*: Soil, Water, Plant and feed
(c) *Activity*: Organisms synthesize a visions policy cucharide in citerical it heat forms slime leyes or capsule on cell, Milk favours formation of capsules in citerical; sterile skimmed milk is frequently used as culture medium when capsule formation is sought.

(D) Biochemical Type IV Protocolytic

(a) *Example*: Bacillus spp. like *B. sublies, B. Cercus.*
   Source: Soil, Water and utensils. Also, Pseudonymous spp. like mentioned carlies and also, Proteus spp. and *streptococcus liquefacicus.*

Biochemical Activity

These organism dicyclic casein to pepteicles which may be furthers disinfected to amino acids; Proteolysis may be preceded by coagulation of cusein by enzyme renin. The end products of proteolysis may in part abnormal flavour or odious to milk.

(E) Lipolytic organisms (Biochemical Type V)

(a) *Examples*: Pseudonymous flavour *Achromobacter lipolyticum, Candidli polytica* and Penicillium spp.
(b) *Source*: Soil, water and utensils
(c) *Activity*: They hydrolyse milk fats to glycerol and fatty acids; some fatty acids imports rancid odour and flavour to milk.

(5) Micrococci

(a) *Example*: *Micrococcus luteus, M. varians, M. freudenreichii* etc.
(b) *Source*: Ducts to cows mammary glands dairy utensils etc.
(c) *Activity*: The small amount of lactic acid is produced (weakly fermentive). also weakly proteolytic, moderately heat resistant, i.e. some strain are capable of surviving at 63°C for 30 minutes.

Classified of Milk Microbes according to Temperature Characteristics, i.e., Temperature Response: Growth and biochemical activities of bacteria in milk large by depends temperature available. They require optimum temperature for growth and activities. Low temperature are used to prevent changes by microbes, and high temperature to reduce their population and kill pathogenic bacteria.

(1) Psychropilic

Grow at temperature above freezing and refrigeration temperature (*i.e.* 4-5°C), produces spoilage effect resulting in 'off' flavour and odours, although low temperature is recommended for prevention of milk, e.g. pseudonyms, Achromobacter, Vibri, Favobacterium and Alcoligenes genera. They are killed by pasteurization, but sometimes even found in pasteurized milk also. The contamination after pasteurization is by equipment, cow bettles etc.

(2) Mesophilic microbes

Grow at moderate temperature *e.g.* 37-39°C, *e.g.*, streptococci, Lactobacilli and coliform, produced acid, gas and off flavours, can be killed by pasteurization process.

(3) Thermophilic bacteria

Grow well at temperature used in pasteurization, i.e., 62°C, but if milk is held at this temperature for 30 minutes, they are destroyed, e.g. Bacillus and clostridium, but bacillus, sterothermophilus even grow at 65°C.

(4) Thermoduir

Are these which survive at pasteurization process but do not grow at pasteurization temperature. They are extremely trouble some as not killed by pasteurization, they contaminate and accumulate as result of improves cleaning of equipment. Therefore subsequent batches of milk is heavily contaminated.

Example

Microbacterium lactium, Micrococcus luteus, Streptococcus and *Bacillus subtilis* etc.

Classification and types of milk organisms on basis of ability to cause infection or disease

Recently Studied that a number of infection are of milk bevibillness, therefore, both bovine and human pathogens isolated from milk; it may leads to number of epidermics, but due to good sanitation reduced. The micobe can be derived either from cattle itself humans involved or milking process etc.

A variety of diseases transmitted from cattle: Human beings e.g. = T.B. Bruceltosis (causing cobortion), salmonellosis foods and mouth disease, and, fever caused by *Coxille burneti* (infecting lungs). streptococcus pyogenes etc., serrate fever trashes on skin caused by streptococcus spp.

These infected cattle but sometimes also to human beings.

These enters directly into milk from udder or in from of body discharge like drops or splashes etc. and cause infection to human beings.

Some diseases are human origin and man-cattle of man, e.g. typhoid fever, diptheria, dysentery, septic, sour-throat, serrate fever, peliomyels are infections spreading from man. Man (inflammation of udder caused by staphylococcus aurcus). The infecting organisms in some cares has been traced to humans. The most common problems due to infected food and milk in human is gastrointestinal troubles etc. Hence, proper hygienic conditions and preservative of milk is necessary to minimize pathogenic contamination of the milk and its products.

Microbiological Examination of Milk

If milk is all allowed to stand for sometime, at room temperature, a large number of microbes develops from the initial inoculum introduced by contaminating. The number of microbes present at time of consumption is determined by the following factors:

1. The temperature at which milk is kept.
2. Time interval between production and consumption.
3. Amount of initial microbes present.
4. Weather milk is pasteurized or not.

Various microbiological and chemical Tests are made to certain proper handling. Treatment and sanitation of milk, high microbial count does not mean that is contains pathogenic microbes: but only indicates excessive contamination. The total mesophilic plate counts are widely used as indicators of milk and its products quality. The examination is also necessary to test presence of pathogenic organisms and spoilage of milk.

Recently a look for indicator organism for monitoring quality of milk and other food products have been developed. A good quality indicator organism is always present in enough numbers. When a pathogen is present so as to easily detected for, e.g. *E. coli*, normal flora of cut is used. But is also has certain limitation, e.g. if Salmonella etc. are present *E. coil* number more acts as indicator organism.

The examination of milk and its products also depends on types of labs, e.g. government labs make tests to as certain public health standards. The food plant labs of quality control tests raw products and ingredients as a warning of possible troubles in manufacture of products. Private control agencies tests to enable the recommendation or acceptance of typical brand of food or milk products. Labs of commercial control agencies, e.g. American daily milk institute may set the standards described and describes desirable or recommend methods of examination.

Some important methods of milk examination:

Standards Plate Count Methods (SPC)

It is enumeration method for examination of milk. In this agar plates are commonly used for estimation of number of bacteria in milk. In a normal routine lab, the most sensitive method detecting presence of a viable bacterium is allow it amplify itself to form a visible colony. It forms basis of traditional pour plate, spread plate or miler and misra drop plate still widely used in microbiological labs.

The normal procedure of this method is to prepare a number of sufficient serial dilution of milk. One ml of diluted sample is mixed with melted agar at 45°C, and the inoculated mediums is then peured into the petriplate. The plate are incubated 32°C-35°C for 48 hrs. for normal routine work at 7°C 7-10 days prychrophiles or at 55°C for 48 hrs. for enumeration of thermophil. Their the number of visible colonies are counted and the number of colonies per ml of milk is reported as spc of given sample. But sometime 45°C Agar destroys psychrophilic 'Spread plate is beneficial because it provides well aerobic environment but sample size should be small 0.1 ml.

In a thoroughly mixed microbes the number of propagules forming colonies are expected to have a poison distribution a property of which is that variance is equal to mean, i.e.

$$X = var = S^2 \tag{1}$$

A consequence of this is that limiting procession of a colony count is dependent on number colonies counted. The 95% confidence limits (cl) can be estimated as approximately.

$$2s = 2x \sqrt{x} \tag{2}$$

(If x is count, on signal plate and has to be our estimate of mean). Thus, for a plate only with 16 colonies the 95% cl would be approximately - 50% (i.e. we have 95% confidence that count lies between 8 to 24).

For plates count, the plates most be over-crowdal. The 30-300 colonies are considered as appropriate dilution is essential. A commonly used dilute known as maximum recovery diluent contains 0.1% peptone and 0.85% of sodium chloride.

But traditional plate counts are expensive so, recently plates have been developed. Only a small volume of each dilution (20) is considered. A number of dilutions can be grow on a single plate. It saves about 2/3 of material as time required colonies after incubation are counted in special grid.

The usual media used in plate count agar but various other selective media are also used for specific microbes.

Advantage of plate count method: The method is very easily and can be used as a routine examination method for estimation of number of bacteria in milk for milk quality. In England and Wales, the milk marketing Board (MMB) introduced in 1982 used such methods and accordingly, flavour are made payment for products or even penalty them.

Disadvantage of plant count method

1. For proper plate count each microbial all should be well separated, but in milk, a number of microbes may be in form of dumps or clusters. Thus, single colony produced may misguide about count.
2. All microbes do not grows in a particular physical environment and media.
3. Some rapidly growing microbes inhibits growth of other microbes.

Thus, SPC is only 'estimation' and bot the total actual count of bacteria in milk.

Direct Microscopic count (DMC) Method

For examination of milk and other food products the possibility of detecting the microbes directly under microscopic should not be missed. The microbial content of milk is determined by direct examination under a microscope by preparing a smear. The producer of this examination is as follows:

The smear is prepared by spreading exactly 0.01 ml of milk on area of 1cm^2 by means of sterile pipette or sysynge. The smear is air dried and stained with solution of methylene blue now, the slide is examined under oil emission objective (100x) for the estimation of microbial of density. Now final count is estimated as follow:

The diameter of most oil emission leusa is 0.16 mm. Thus, area seen under oil emission is calculated as πr^2 (i.e., 3.14 × (0.85)^2 = 0.02 mm^2 new smear is prepared on area of 1 cm^2 or = 100 mm^2: There would be 100/0.02, i.e. 500 fields. The average count of one field is multiplied by total number of fields. This will gave the total number of microbes in 0.01 ml of milk samples.

The numerous large clumps of bacterial indicate uncleaned utensils many Puss cells indicates infected workers. The streptococci indicates possible mastitis. It is common practice to report result in turns of dump counts. The method is applied to mainly unpasteurized milks as heating causes many bacteria to loose their staining properties.

Advantage of DMC

1. The method of more rapid and takes only about 15 minutes. Thus, a large number of samples can be examined.
2. Only limited equipments required.
3. The slides can be kept for permanent records and examination whenever required.
4. Different morphological; type can be easily distinguished in slid preparations. This is of great value for determining source and nature of contamination.

Disadvantages

1. The count is not applicable if number of microbes is low in milk. Because a large factor is used for converting number of organism per field to the number per ml of milk.
2. The method is not applicable to differentiate between living (viable) and non-living microbes.
3. It could not be used for pasteurized milk because most of organism are dead except this the direct epifloursent filter technique (DEFT) is a microscopic technique was developed for estimating bacterial counts in raw milk. It was developed for testing hygienic quality of from milk. It involves concentration of large number of microbes from a higher volume of sample by filtering through poly carbonate membrane filter. The retained bactria are stained on the membrane with acridine arrange and counted directing under epiflorescene microscopes. It may be necessary to protect the sample to allow filtration; thus, milk can be pretreated with detergent and pretcure enzyme. It is also necessary that bacteria should be trapped in a single focal plane because of limited depths of focus of the microscopical at the magnifications required.

A cridine orange is meta chromatic fluorochrome flugresing either green or orange. When bond to double standard DNA, it fluorece green and when bond to single standard RNA, it flouresce orange, generally assumed that there cells which fluoresce yellow are viable, while these green are non-viable (not always true).

The actual colour of individual cell largely depends upon concentration of dye within cell. In many microbes in which cell maintains its integety, dye doesn't pass into cell and fleruresce green and many dead cell from which dye leaks in fleruresce orange. This method also found application in examination of meat and fish, meat and fish products. Berverayes and vital microbes on water samples.

Numerical Relationship between Direct and Plate Counts

The direct count is usually five to ten or more times high than plate count because former enumerates individuals, even these in dumps and also dead bacteria. The plate count enumerates only live bacteria capable of developing in the media and at temperature given. Each clump count only as a single bacterium as each cumps contains several dozen of individual cells yet a dump usually yield only one colony.

A comparison of Sensitivity of Methods Umeriatic is shown in Table 2.2.

Qualitative Analysis of Milk and its Products

Reductase Test

As milk is drawn out of cattle it comes in contact with air and acquires an oxidation-reduction potential (X/R) of + 30 mv (Milli Volts). As contamination occurs and microbes starts grow in milk, it causes lowering of X/R potential. The rate of shift of X/R potential depends upon number and kinds of organisms present and their metabolic rate. This forms the basis of reductase test for examination of milk. This shift of X/R potential car e determined by are of various dyes like methylene blue, Resazurin which indicates by their colour change on oxidation.

Table 2.2
Sensitivity of Methods Umeriatic

Method	Vol of sample	Count (cfu/ml)
Direct Microscopy	5×10^6	2×10^6
Miles and micra	0.02	2×10^2
Spread plate	0.1	10^2
Pour plate	1.0	10
MPN	3×10.0	0.10
	4.3×1	
	4.3×0.1	

Many redox reactions involve the transfer of O_2. One reactant may acts as e^- donar and other as e^- acceptor. Thus, rate at which the suostrate (milk) is oxidized by living organisms. It is a rapid method of examination for manufacturing of milk and its products and is also cost effected.

(1) MBRT or Methylene Blue Reductase Test

It is based on the principle that dye is coloured when oxidized, but colourless when it is reduced. For this test, 10 ml of milk sample is pipetted into a sterile-tube and ml of standard methylene blue solution (final content: 1 : 300,000) is added. The tube is closed with a rubber stopper and inverted 3 times to mix. It is plaud at 35.5°C in water bath immediately. The tube is inverted after every one hours for colours test and examined after every 30 minutes until decolouization occurs. The result is reported in terns of time required for reduction of methylene blue. The reduction time is inversely proportional to the initial microbial content. When number of microbes is more O/R potential is more and dye is reduced due to rapid consumption of O_2 by microbes.

(2) Resazurium Reductase Test

Now-a-days, another dye Resazurin is used for reductase test it undergoes a series of colour change depending upon O/R potential. Thus, this dye permits readings of degree of reduction of short intervals them does methylene blue. It undergoes a serial change from slate blue to pink to colourless.

Table 2.3
Methylene Blue Reductase Test Time and the Quality of Milk

MBRT Time	Quality of milk
30 minutes	very poor
30 min-2hr	poor
2 hr-6hr	fair
5 hr-5hr	good
More than 8hr	excellent

The test is performed by mixing 1.20000 dilution of 1ml of resazurin to 10 ml of milk sample in a sterile tube and kept at water bath at 35-37°. The colour change sequence is as below:

Slate blue → Pink blue → Pink → Decolourize

There are two methods employed for this reduction test.

(a) One hours test method

One ml of dye is added to 10ml of milk in sterile tube and stand for 1 hour 37°C temperature. New colour of milk is compared to already prepared standard solution of different colours mentioned earlier.

It colour change	Quality
Gr I slate blue → Pink blue	Good, less no. of microbes
Gr II slate blue → Marve	Higher mircobial content
Gr III statable pink → Pink	Growly by abnormal
Gr IV statable colourless → pink	Highly contaminated

Gr IV, the milk may contain many puss cells, and is probably teeming with mastitis organisms.

(b) Three Hours Test

In this same principal is employed and reading were taken at 3 times at 1 hour intervals. High grade milk requires at dert 3 hours for decolourization. The reading is reported as resazurin reduction time (RRT).

From 1937 and until recently, MBRT was a statutory test for grading milk quality in England and Wales, changes in technology, especially refrigeration has made this test less reliable because it shows little correlation with psychrophilic bacteria. As reduction of resazurin takes place in two stages of colours there is wider range of colour that can be scored by using standard computer disc within less time thus,

Resozurin →	Resofurin →	Di hydroresofurin
(Blue)	(Pink)	(Leuco)
Oxidized	Intermediate	Reduced.

3

KHOA PRODUCTS

Milk is an excellent medium for the growth of micro-organism. The odour of milk is due to the activity of the milk organisms. Milk can be contaminated from the udder to the vessels. Good hygienic conditions are to be used on all levels of milk handling to keep the bacterial count level low. However, the quality of milk can also be preserved by concentrating milk into products, like *khoa*, condensed milk, milk powder etc. Just to further increase the storage life of *khoa*, sugar is added and sweet like *burfi*, *peda*, lodge etc., are prepared. Thus, by adding sugar not only the storage life of *khoa* is increased but palatability is also improved. However, the manner in which these products are sold in the market are liable to be contaminated by all sort of micro-organism. Therefore, we were planned to know the microbiological and chemical quality of *burfi*, *peda* and lodge sold on *halwai* shops in the local market.

Collection of Samples

We collected samples of *peda*, *lodge*, *burfi* and chemical and micribiological tests should be done in the Lab. Sample of *burfi*, *peda* and lodge collected from the market were either from show cases or from open pans. Hence, in all ten samples of each products (*burfi*, *peda* and lodge) were collected, therefore, in total thirty samples were analysed.

The collected *burfi*, *peda* and lodge were analysed for chemical tests like moisture, fat, ash sugar and protein percentage. Microbiological tests consists of S.P.C. MPN, spore, yeast and mold and pathogens counts.

(A) Chemical Analysis

1. Moisture Percentage

Moisture Percentage of *Khoa* based sweets, was determined by drying in the oven at 90°C for 2 hours moisture percentage was calculated as follows:

Weigh of Petridish	=	W1 g
Weigh of petridish and Dried product	=	W2 g
Weigh of moisture in 10 g of product	=	10 – (W2 – W1)
Moisture Percentage	=	10 – (W2 – W1) × 100/10

2. Fat Percentage

Fat was determined by gravimetric method:

Rose Gottieb Method: Five grams of sample of *khoa* based sweets 10 ml of water added to the sample are transferred to an extraction apparatus and 1 ml of concentrated ammonia solution added. After mixing 10ml ethyl alcohol the mixture is vigorously shaken for 1 minutes and then 25 ml diethyl ether added and shaking repeated for one minutes then 25 ml petroleum ether is added shaking repeated. After standing for at list 30 minutes the clear layer is separated and extraction repeated twice. The combined ethereal extracts are evaporated and the fat weighted.

3. Ash Percentage

Ash Percentage of *Khoa* based sweets was determined by burying a known quantity of the product (10 g) in Silica crucible till it is converting into whitish colour ash. Ash Percentage was calculated as follows:

Weight of Silica crucible	=	W1 g
Weight of Silica crucible + burnt product	=	W2 g
Weight of Ash in	=	10 – (W2 – W1) g

10 g of product

Ash Percentage $= 10 - (W2 - W1) \times 100/10$

4. *Sugar percentage*

Sucrose does not reduce fehling solution, but on hydrolysis (called inversion of sucrose) is changed into reducing sugar such as glucose and fructose in equimolecular quantities.

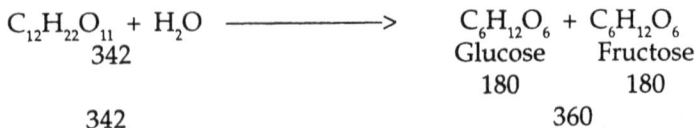

$$C_{12}H_{22}O_{11} + H_2O \longrightarrow C_6H_{12}O_6 + C_6H_{12}O_6$$

$$342 \hspace{4cm} \text{Glucose} \quad \text{Fructose}$$

$$\hspace{4.5cm} 180 \hspace{1.5cm} 180$$

$$342 \hspace{4cm} 360$$

Therefore, One gram reducing sugar $= 342/360$

$\hspace{6.7cm} = 0.95$ g sucrose

The inverted sugar was titrated

Against fehling solution sucrose $=$ Reducing sugar

$\hspace{7cm} \times 0.95$

PROCEDURE

We take 5 or 6 grams of *khoa* based sample was taken and dissolved in distilled water. The mixture was transferred into 100 ml volumetric flask. Finally the volume was made up with the help of distilled water.

Twenty-five ml of this 5 per cent solution was transferred to 250 ml of volumetric flask using 25 ml pipette. After adding 25 ml of distilled water and 5 ml of 60% HCl the flask was heated in such a way that the temperature rises 68°C in 10 minute and kept it at this temperature for another 5 minutes. Then the thermometer was removed. The stem and the bulb of thermometer were washed into the flask with water. A piece of litmus paper was placed into the flask and neutralized the inverted sugar by adding 5% sodium hydroxide and the volume was made up. The contents were shaken well to got a homogeneous solution.

The solution was taken in burette and titrated against hot 10 ml fehling solution plus 10 ml of distilled water. During titration the flask was kept over burner in order to keep it hot. Sugar solution was added gradually (2.0 ml at a time) till the reddish colour appears. Then three drops of methylene blue indicator was added and titration continued till, the permanent brick red colour appears. Finally the reading was noted. Percentage of sugar was calculated as follows:

Supposed 20 ml or the actual amount
of the invert sugar used up in
titration   = 20 ml
Strength of solution   = 56 g/litre
10ml fehling solution neutralize   = 0.50 g glucose
Therefore, 0.50 gm glucose   = 20 ml invert sugar
Weight of glucose in 250 ml
of invert sugar   = (250 * 0.50)/20
                                             = 0.635 g

This (0.625 g) amount is actually present in 25 ml of sugar solution.

Glucose is 100 ml sugar   = $\dfrac{100 \times 0.625}{25}$

1 g reducing sugar   = 0.95 g sucrose
2.5 g glucose   = 2.5 × 0.95
                                             = 2.375 g sucrose

Sucrose % in sample   = $\dfrac{100 \times 2.375}{5}$

                                             = 4.75%
Sucrose in (*Bura*) was calculated   = 90%
90 g sucrose is present in   = 100 g *bura*
1 g sucrose is present in   = 100/90 g *bura*

47.5 g sucrose is present in   = $\dfrac{100 \times 47.5}{90}$

                                             = 52.77% (*bura*)

5. Protein Percentage

Protein was determined by difference.
Protein Percentage =   100 − (moisture + Fat
                             + Ash + Sugar Percentage)

B. Microbiological Analysis

Microbiological analysis was done according to ISI (Indian Standard Institution) standard methods given as follows:

1. Standard Plate Count (S.P.C.)

The S.P.C. suggested by Indian Standard Institution is followed:

Standard Plate Count of *Khoa* based sweet was determined on standard milk agar and the product dilutions were prepared in normal physiological saline solution (0.9% NaCl in distilled water). Dilutions vary from 10^{-2}, 10^{-4}. The plates were incubated at a temperature $37 \pm 1°C$ for 72 hours and the colonies were counted. The total count was determined after multiplying with dilution used. So the total number of organisms per gram were determined.

2. Spore Count

The spore count of products was determined in nutrient agar, product dilutions were prepared in normal physiological saline solution (0.9% NaCl in distilled water). Dilution was $10.2\text{-}10^{-4}$. Saline solution having test product in it was heated at 161°F for 30 seconds to kill all the vegetative cells. It was then diluted to 10^{-4} and then plated. The plates were incubated at $37 \pm 1°C$ for 72 hours and the viable count was determined.

3. Coliform Count

For counting the coliform organisms in food pour plate method was used. Violet red bile salt agar was the solidifiable media used in this method.

The product dilutions were prepared in normal physiological saline solution.

Dilution vary from 10^{-2} to 10^{-3}. The violet red bile salt agar was melted and cooled to 45°C, mixed well for 72 hours. After incubation the number of colonies were counted. The colonies were dark red having about 0.5 mm diameter.

4. Yeast and Mold

Yeast and mould counts were determined on potato dextrose agar. Product dilution were prepared in normal physiological saline solution. Dilutions vary from 10^{-2} to 10^{-3} 1.0 ml lactic acid (10.0%) was added in the medium before finally adding to petric disc to bring down its pH to a desirable level. The plates were incubated at temperature of 25 to 1°C for 72 hours and the viable count was determined.

5. Pathogenic Count

Pathogenic count was determined in staphylococcal medium–110. Product dilution were prepared in normal physiological saline solution, dilutions very from 10^{-2} to 10^{-4}. The plates were incubated at a temperature of 37 $\pm$ 1°C for 72 hours and viable count were determined.

Results and Discussion

Nutritional qualities of surplus milk are conserved by dehydrating it into *khoa* or *mawa*. This dehydrated milk product has the longer shelf life than milk, but it is hardly consumed by consumers as such because it is hardly consumed by consumers as such because it is not very much palatable. So, with *mawa* sugar (*bura* – crude sucrose form) is mixed and some heat treatment is given to it. It improves its palatability as well as its shelf life. Therefore, product like *burfi, peda,* lodge, *kalakand,* etc. are prepared on *halwai* shops by mixing sugar to *mawa.* All these *mawa* based sweets have *mawa* plus sugar in different proportions but they differ in their heat treatment definitely. This results in variation of texture, flavour and composition of these products.

Those products are regularly sold on *halwai* shops in open in closed show cases. This difference in display of *Mawa* based sweets definitely cause difference in their microbiological quality.

Therefore, this study was planned to know the chemical and Microbiological quality of these milk products displayed in open pans and in show cases on *halwai* shops. For this purpose *burfi, peda* and lodge samples (10 each totaling 30 sample) were

collected from local market and immediately brought to Dairy
Laboratory for analysis.

SAMPLES

Open Plan		Show Case	
1.	*Chemical Composition*	*2.*	*Chemical Composition*
(a)	Moisture percentage	*(a)*	Moisture Percentage
(b)	Fat Percentage	*(b)*	Fat Percentage
(c)	Ash Percentage	*(c)*	Ash Percentage
(d)	Sugar Percentage	*(d)*	Sugar Percentage
(e)	Protein	*(e)*	Protein
2.	*Microbiological Test*	*2.*	*Microbiological Tests*
(a)	SPC	*(a)*	SPC
(b)	Spare Count	*(b)*	Spare Count
(c)	Coliform count	*(c)*	Coliform count
(d)	Y*(d)*	Y	
(e)	Pathogenic count	*(e)*	Pathogenic Count

The results so obtained were statistically treated and tabulated
in Table 3.1 to Table 3.8.

Chemical Composition

1. Moisture Percentage

Moisture percentage in the product definitely affects the shelf
life of the product, and shelf life is further enhanced by the
addition of sugar to it. Amount of moisture also change the body
and texture of the product which is typical for a particular product
sold in the market. Sometimes moisture is also adjusted to earn
more profit. Consequently the Government fixes the supper limit
of moisture permissible in the product and beyond this the *halwai*
or hawker is liable to be prosecuted.

Hence, moisture percentage of every sample was determined,
statistically treated and tabulated in Table 3.1.

It is clear from Table 3.1 that the average moisture percentage
(11.83) is lowest for *burfi* samples, not only this, the minimum
(8.10) and the maximum (14.30) values are also lowest in all the
three products in question. Next comes *peda* and lastly (highest)

comes lodge. Although the average moisture percentage is lower in *peda* than yet the highest percentage of moisture in the same (17.10) in both the products (*peda* and lodge). The samples of *peda* have got highest variation (10.75-17.10), S.D. value 2.14, but more values are close to the minimum value consequently the over all average was lower than lodge. The S.D. value of lodge is quite low (1.62) which indicates the uniformity in its production resulting in uniform chemical composition.

Table 3.1
The amount of Moisture in different samples of burfi, peda and lodge procured from local market

Sample No.	Burfi	Peda	Lodge
1	8.10	12.60	14.00
2	11.20	16.20	16.35
3	12.60	10.75	11.80
4	14.00	16.00	16.00
5	13.40	14.30	12.80
6	10.50	11.50	15.60
7	13.20	11.60	13.60
8	11.25	12.40	13.80
9	14.30	17.10	17.10
10	9.80	13.20	15.40
Minimum	8.10	10.75	11.80
Maximum	14.30	17.10	17.10
Average	11.83	13.56	14.72
S.D.	1.90	2.14	1.62

Date and Bhatia (1955) for *burfi*, Ghodekar (1969) for both *peda* and *burfi*, Vijayabhadar et al. (1983) and Choudary (1985) for *peda* have reported lower percentage of moisture than the values reported in this study. Hemavathy *et al.* (1977), Shama and Zariwala (1978), Mandokhot et al. (1985), Rajorhia and Sen (1987) have given a wide variation than given in this study. But Dwarakanath and Srikant (1977) for *burfi*, Patel (1986) for *peda* have given the similar results. Sachdeva and Rajorhia (1982) have also given the similar range of values as given in the investigation. Singh (1986) has reported highest moisture percentage in lodge, while *burfi* and *peda* have the same percentage of moisture.

So on the basis of moisture percentage we can place *burfi*, *peda* and lodge in ascending order.

2. Fat Percentage

Fat percentage is a very important constituent of these sweets, i.e., *burfi*, *peda* and lodge. As it gives a better body and texture to the finished product and also improves its flavour and taste. It is a good source of energy as well. Hence, every sample of sweet was analysed for fat gravimetrically by Rose Gottlieb method. The results obtained are presented in Table 3.2 after they are treated statistically.

Table 3.2
The amount of Fat in different samples of burfi, peda and lodge procured from local market

Sample No.	Burfi	Peda	Lodge
1	17.00	22.20	19.20
2	18.20	24.00	21.20
3	21.00	28.10	24.00
4	16.20	19.70	28.80
5	19.40	27.20	34.00
6	17.20	25.20	27.20
7	18.00	19.20	26.00
8	21.20	27.20	33.60
9	16.80	26.20	28.20
10	14.00	18.20	20.30
Minimum	14.00	18.20	19.20
Maximum	21.20	28.10	34.00
Average	17.90	23.72	26.25
S. D.	2.08	3.33	4.91

On the perusal of Table 3.2 we find that the lowest fat percentage is reported for *burfi* along with lowest range of value (14.00-21.20) S.D. Values 2.08. The highest fat percentage with highest variation (S.D. Value 4.91) is reported for lodge samples. And the *peda* samples come in between *burfi* and lodge. Therefore, we can say that lodge is quire rich nutritionally and *burfi* is comparatively poor in nutritional qualities.

When we compare the results of present work with that of given in literature we find a great variation. Garg *et al.* (1984) and Patel (1986) gave similar percentage of fat for *peda* while nearly all workers reported lower values of fat in *peda* and *burfi*.

Date and Bhatia (1955) for *Burfi*, ghodekar for *burfi* and *peda*, Hemavathy *et al.* (1974), Zariwala (1978) for *burfi* and Ipeda Sachdeva and Rajarhia for *burfi* and Rajarhia and Sen (1987) for *burfi* and *peda*, all gave lower value of fat.

Therefore, we can place lodge, *Peda* and *burfi* in the descending order on the basis of fat content and nutritionally, they will be grated in the same order.

3. Ash Percentage

The amount to Ash in *burfi*, *peda* and lodge indirectly indicate the amount of *mawa* used in the manufacture of the product. Because in the burning of the sweets all fats, all sugar all moisture and nearly are protein are burnt to no ash because there are the organic substances having C, H and O only. Except few proteins which have ash material in fat. Therefore, ash was also determined in all the sample of *burfi*, *peda* and lodge. The result are tabulated in Table 3.3 after proper statistical treatment.

Table 3.3
The amount of Ash in different samples of burfi, peda and lodge procured from local market

Sample No.	Burfi	Peda	Lodge
1	3.2	3.8	3.8
2	3.4	3.4	2.9
3	4.5	4.1	2.0
4	3.7	2.9	1.6
5	2.8	3.1	2.0
6	2.5	2.5	2.4
7	1.2	1.3	1.5
8	1.4	1.2	1.8
9	1.5	4.8	2.1
10	1.9	2.4	2.4
Maximum	1.2	1.2	1.5
Maximum	4.5	4.8	3.8
Average	2.6	2.9	2.2
S. D	1.06	1.26	0.802

It is clear from Table 3.3 that average ash percentage is highest (2.9%) in *peda*. *Peda* samples also have the highest variation (1.2-4.8) which is clear from S.D. value (1.26). While lodge has got the minimum (2.2) ash percentage and minimum variation (1.5-3.8) as well as it is also clear from S.D. value (0.802) for lodge which is lowest in all the three product. So on the basis of ash percentage we can place *peda*, *burfi* and lodge in the descending order.

Hemvathy (1974), and Rajorhia and Sen (1987) have given higher range of ash values for *burfi* and *peda*. However, Ghedekar (1969) have given lower average ash percentage for *burfi* and *peda*, similarly Vijayabhode *et al.* (1983) have given lower ash percentage for market as well as laboratory prepared *peda*.

Date and Bhatia (1955), collected *burfi* samples from market and reported average 2.6 per cent ash in these *burfi* samples. The result of data and Bhatia are quite in agreement with the result of present study (Table 3.3)

So, in the end we can say that sample have the highest average value of ash as well as highest variation in values. However, lodge has got the lowest average ash value as well as lowest variation between minimum and maximum (1.5-3.8) values, S.D. Value 0802. *Burfi* comes in between.

4. Sugar percentage

Addition of sugar to *Mawa* is a normal feature in the preparation of sweets. It's purpose is to improve palatability. Not only this is also preserves *Mawa* for some longer period. Sometime the addition of sugar to *mawa* has a objective to earn profit from sweets. This objective may not be kept in mind always. However, sometimes (mainly in mela's) it is determined in this study.

Results of sugar analysis are presented in Table 3.4. It is clear from this table that sugar percentage is minimum (27.45%) of lodge. Sugar percentage of lodge also have the minimum variation (22.51-35.98). S. D. value 4.18, while the maximum sugar percentage (45.47) is used for *burfi*, but it dose not have the maximum variation (32.68-58.22), S.D. 8.32. Sugar percentage in *peda* comes in between lodge and *burfi* (39.51) but the variation is highest (26.84-54.91), S.D. 9.53. It means that the technique of lodge preparation is almost standardized. Another reason may

Table 3.4

The Amount of Sugar in different samples of burfi, peda and lodge procured from local market

Sample No.	Burfi			Peda			Lodge		
	B.R (ml)	Sucrose	Bura	B.R. (ml)	Sucrose	Bura	B. R. (ml)	Sucrose	Bura
1.	18.6	50.92	56.57	24.2	39.25	43.61	26.4	35.98	39.98
2.	22.0	43.42	48.13	22.0	43.18	47.97	30.0	31.66	35.18
3.	28.2	33.44	37.15	31.5	30.15	33.50	38.7	24.55	27.27
4.	19.2	49.40	54.88	21.8	43.57	48.82	35.5	26.76	29.73
5.	25.4	37.24	41.37	35.4	26.84	29.81	42.2	22.51	25.00
6.	28.6	32.68	36.31	33.2	28.61	31.79	38.4	24.74	27.49
7	18.6	50.92	56.57	18.4	51.63	57.37	26.6	25.95	28.84
8.	21.2	44.84	49.82	17.3	54.91	61.00	41.2	23.05	25.62
9.	16.2	58.52	65.02	31.0	30.65	34.05	34.6	27.46	30.51
10.	17.8	53.37	59.30	20.5	46.34	51.00	29.8	31.88	35.42
Minimum		32.68	36.31		26.84	29.81		22.51	25.00
Maximum		58.52	65.02		54.91	61.00		35.98	39.98
Average		45.47	50.51		39.51	43.90		27.45	30.50
S. D.		8.32	9.23		9.53	10.59		4.18	8.86

be that only few *halwai*'s are preparing it and so they are following their own techniques for it preparation.

In literature only the results of *burfi* and *peda* analysis are available, however, nobody has so far given result for lodge for *burfi* the following Results have been given in percentage by different workers. Date and Bhatia (1955) 54.3 and Ghedekar (1969) 52.0 have reporter a higher percentage of sugar in *burfi* but Dwarakanath and Srikanta (1977) 40.80; Garg *et al.* (1984) 29; Choudhary (1985) 32.71 all have given the lower percentage of sugar in *burfi*. Workers like Hemavathy *et al.* (1974); Shama and Zariwala (1978) 16.7 to 59.7; Sachdeva and Rajorhia (1982) 26.0 to 58.0; Mandokhot *et al.* (1985) 16.7 to 59.7 and Rajorhia and sen (1987) 24.8 to 59.7 have given a wide variation in sugar percentage of *burfi*.

For *peda* the following results have been given in literature. Ghodekar *et al.* (1969) 55.3; Dwarkanath and Srikanta (1974) 59.4 and Vijaybhader *et al.* (1983) 63.50; have reported a higher percentage of sugar in *peda*, but Garg *et al.* (1984) 29.0; Choudhary (1985) 34.63 and Patel (1998) 31.8 all have given the lower percentage of sugar in *peda*. Workers like Mandokhot *et al.* (1985) 13.2 to 61.8 and Rajorhia and Sen (1987) 24.8 to 54.2 have given a wide variation in sugar percentage of *peda*.

Singh (1986) has given 27.74 percent sugar in lodge which is quite similar to results of present work (27.45).

Therefore, we can place lodge, *peda* and *burfi* in an ascending order on the basis of sugar percentage.

5. Protein Percentage

Protein are not only important but essential in human diet. The proteins of animal organ are still essential to get all the essential amino acids in diet. Milk proteins are the only source of these essential amino acids in the diet of a vegetarian in India. Therefore, we always try to get milk and milk products included in the diet of vegetarians in India. From nutritional point of view it becomes essential to include protein determination in *burfi*, *peda* and lodge. The protein percentage in these products was determined by difference = 100 − (Moisture + Ash + Fat + Sugar) = Protein. The results so obtained were tabulated in Table 3.5, and statistically treated.

On the basis of sewage result presented in any food material, Therefore, this test is also know as viable count. This test is very widely used to determine the number and type of organisms found in milk and milk products. Therefore, this test was also applied in this investigation. The results of this test are presented in Table 3.6.

Table 3.5
The amount of Protein in different samples of burfi, peda and lodge procured from local market

Sample No.	Burfi	Peda	Lodge
1	20.78	22.15	27.02
2	23.78	13.22	28.89
3	28.46	26.90	37.65
4	16.70	17.83	26.84
5	27.16	28.56	28.69
6	37.12	32.19	30.06
7	16.68	16.27	32.15
8	21.31	4.29	27.75
9	9.88	21.25	25.14
10	20.93	19.86	20.02
Minimum	9.88	4.29	20.02
Maximum	37.12	32.19	37.65
Average	22.98	20.25	28.42
S. D.	4.84	7.66	6.96

It is clear from Table 3.6 that this lowest average count (8.7 × 10^4/g) was found in *burfi*. Not only the count is lowest in *burfi*, but the range is also lowest) 2-20.5 × 10^4/g) as apparent from SD value (5.984). Peculiarly enough *peda* sample given highest SPC (17.1 × 10^4/g) and also highest variation (2-39.5 × 10^4/g). This highest count is due to very poor quality of sample No. 3 and 7. If we exclude these two samples then the average SPC count don to 12.5 × 10^4/g only. So we can say that the SPC of *Peda* sample are definite lower than lodge however due to the poor quality of *peda* sample the result give misleading inference. Actually these two samples are taken from shop where *peda* is displayed in open pan. The average SPC value and rang for lodge come in between *burfi* and *peda*.

Table 3.6
The Standard Plate Count in different samples of burfi, peda and lodge procured from local market

Sample No.	Burfi (10^4)	Peda (10^4)	Lodge (10^4)
1	3.0	5.0	4.0
2	4.0	7.5	21.0
3	13.5	31.5	6.0
4	2.0	2.0	6.0
5	3.5	17.5	12.0
6	11.0	23.0	7.5
7	8.0	39.5	18.0
8	5.5	4.0	15.5
9	16.0	17.0	23.5
10	20.5	24.0	21.5
Minimum	2.0	2.0	4.0
Maximum	20.5	39.5	23.5
Average	8.7	17.1	13.5
S. D.	5.984	11.962	6.967

In literature also the difference is observed such as Ghodekar *et al.* (1974), Singh *et al.* (1975). Garg *et al.* (1984), Choudhary (1985) and Mandokhot and Garg (1985) all have reported lower S.P.C. for *burfi* and higher for *peda*. Although the result are variable yet the inference is the same. However, Lavania and Gautam (1987) reported higher S.P.C. for *burfi* than *peda* and lodge.

Singh (1986), and Lavania and Gautam (1987) have reported higher standard plate count (26.30 × 10^4 and 16.38 × 10^4 respectively) for lodge than reported in present investigation (13.5 × 10^4).

Therefore, on the basis of SPC we can place *peda*, lodge and *burfi* in descending order.

2. Spore Count

Sporing organisms are capable of surviving high temperature and as such are problem for sweets which are prepared out of *khoa*. While preparing sweets, *khoa* is heated and then sugar is added. Therefore, all the vegetative cells are destroyed, however, spores survive. Therefore, to know the number of spores present indicates the poor quality of ingredients and/or insufficient heating of *khoa*. Therefore, this test was also used in this investigation. The results are resented in Table 3.7.

Table 3.7
The Spore Count in different samples of burfi, peda and lodge procured from local market

Sample No.	Burfi (10^3)	Peda (10^3)	Lodge (10^3)
1	7.0	8.0	29.0
2	15.5	15.0	43.0
3	41.5	111.5	21.5
4	32.5	30.5	6.0
5	20.0	13.5	4.0
6	30.0	26.0	39.0
7	13.0	62.0	44.0
8	12.0	14.0	66.0
9	28.5	16.0	77.0
10	34.0	37.0	44.0
Minimum	7.0	8.0	4.0
Maximum	41.5	111.5	77.0
Average	23.4	33.3	37.3
S.D.	10.834	30.129	22.292

It is clear from this table that the lowest average count (23.4 × 10^3/g) is found in *burfi*. Not only the count is lowest in *burfi*, but the range is also lowest (7.0-41.5/g) as apparent from S.D. value (10.834) also. Lodge samples give highest spore count (37.3 × 10^3/g) but the range is not highest, Fig. 7?? clearly indicate the trend. Range of values have been highest for *peda* (8.0-111.5 × 10^3/g). If we exclude the sample No. 3 (spore count 111.5 × 10^3/g) in *peda* than the average spore count comes down to 24.6 × 10^3/g from 33.3 × 103/g and a very low range is left i.e. 8.0-62.0 only. This range is definite lower than lodge (4.0-77.0 × 10^3/g). Actually this sample No. 3 is taken from the shop of a *halwai* where these sweets are displayed in open pan. Thus this sample is having very high percentage of micro-organisms including spore formers.

In literature Ghodekar *et al.* (1974), Dwarkanath and Srikanta (1977), Choudhary (1985) and Singh (1986) reported lesser number of spore formers in *burfi* and *peda*. But Lavania and Gautam (1987) have reported higher number of spore formers in *burfi*, *peda* and lodge than the number of spores reported in this study. Singh (1986) have reported 21.70×10^3 number of spore formers in lodge which is lower than the present study (37.3×10^3), while Lavalina and Gautam (1987) have reported higher number of spore formers (60.89×10^3) in lodge.

Hence, a lot of variation is found in literature, but in present investigation the results place *burfi*, *peda* and lodge in ascending order.

3. Coliform Count

Coliform organisms are always unwanted in food stuff, as their presence in it indicate the unclean handling of the product. It is also difficult to keep coliform organisms away from the product under Indian conditions. Hence, a maximum limit for coliform count is fixed and it is not more than 10 per gram for *burfi*. Therefore, in this study coliform count was included to know whether the hygienic conditions are followed or not.

In the present investigations all 10 samples of *burfi* and lodge are free from coliform organisms. While only one sample (sample No. 9) of *peda* is positive for coliform count and it gives 1×10^2/ g count.

In literature also some workers have reported absence of coliform organisms in sweets. Kamat and Sulebele (1974) reported no coliform organisms in sweets. Dwarkanath and Srikant (1977) also reported absence of coliform organisms in *burfi*. Similarly Garg *et al.* (1984) could not detect coliform organisms in *burfi* and *peda*, except sample of *peda*. Mandokhot and Garg (1985) have also found some of *burfi* free from coliform organisms.

Therefore, on the basis of coliform test the samples, of *burfi*, *peda* and lodge are judged as good.

So, we can not grade these three product on the basis of this test, as very good. However, the conditions under which the sweets are sold cannot be said very hygienic. Hence, we may say that high sugar percentage in the product caused the destruction of the cells.

4. Yeast and Mould Count

Determination of yeast and moulds count is quite useful for *khoa* and its products, i.e. *burfi, peda* and lodge. Both yeasts and moulds are capable of growing in the medium which are acidic and low in moisture content. Moulds are strict aerobic in nature, therefore, they go only on the surface and cause discolouration on the surface of the product. While yeasts cause internal deterioration of the product. Therefore, yeast and mould count was also included in this study.

In the present investigation all 10 samples of *burfi* and lodge are free from yeasts and moulds. However, only on sample (sample No. 9) of *peda* gives positive results and the count is $3 \times 10^2/g$.

In the literature, mandokhot and Garg (1985) found in Hissar some *burfi* samples free from yeasts and moulds. Similarly Lavania and Gautam (1987) also reported some of the sample of *burfi, peda* and lodge free from yeasts, and some of the sample of lodge free from moulds as well. But all other workers have reported the present of yeasts and moulds in sweets although in verb variable numbers.

This clearly indicates the sale of the products in a well protected manner. Thus avoid any type of external contamination of sweets by yeasts and moulds.

5. Pathogenic Count

Food must always be free from pathogens, their presence is not only unwanted but harmful to consumers as well. Fortunately pathogens are not heat resistance and, therefore, killed when ever food is heated. Hence, we hardly expect any pathogenic organism in these sweets. We hardly expect any pathogenic organism in these sweets. But the way they are sold in the market caused constant contamination of sweets by pathogens. Therefore, pathogenic count was determined in each and every sample of sweets purchased from the market of Baraut. The results are tabulated in Table 3.8, after statistically treated. On the perusal of this Table 3.8, it is apparent that *burfi* samples are having minimum pathogenic count ($6.5 \times 10^2/g$) and also have got the minimum range (3.0-$10.5 \times 10^2/g$). While in lodge the average pathogenic count is highest (15.7 × 10^2/g) and it also has the maximum variation (2.0-40.0 × 10^2/g) as clear from S.D. value 11.10. *Peda* comes in between. The highest pathogenic count in lodge may be due to the two extreme samples Nos. 4 and 7 in which the counts are 28 × 10^2/g) respectively, while in rest of the sample values are less then 17 × 10^2/g. Similarly, in *peda* the sample No. 7 is of extreme value (35.0 × 10^2/g) while other values are 18.0 × 10^2/g or less. Therefore, the extreme value of lodge and *peda* they definitely indicate the unhygienic conditions of display of sweets.

Table 3.8
The Pathogenic Count in different samples of burfi, peda and lodge procured from local market

Sample No.	Burfi (10^2)	Peda (10^2)	Lodge (10^2)
1	5.0	4.0	13.0
2	5.5	6.0	17.0
3	10.5	15.0	11.0
4	4.0	4.5	28.0
5	4.5	15.0	2.0
6	6.5	18.0	15.5
7	3.0	35.0	40.0
8	3.0	Miss (No Colony)	Miss (No Colony)
9	9.5	3.0	5.5
10	7.5	2.5	9.0
Minimum	3.0	2.5	2.0
Maximum	10.5	35.0	40.0
Average	6.5	11.4	15.7
S. D.	1.483	10.097	11.101

One thing is very peculiar in this study that every sample gave positive results, while Gatler *et al.* (1970) have reported the presence of pathogens in 47 per cent samples only. Garg *et al.* (1984) have detected the presence of pathogens in *burfi* as well as in *peda*. Patel (1985) has found Salmonella, Shigella and Staphylococci in open pan sweets. Ranganathan (1984) and Mandokhot and Garg (1985) have reported higher number of pathogens in *burfi* and *peda*, than reported in this investigation.

Therefore, on the basis of pathogenic count *burfi* has the lowest, while lodge the highest and *peda* comes in between.

Comparison of Microbiological quality of *Burfi, Peda* and Lodge displayed and sold in open pans and show cases:

The sweets are always sold on the *halwai* shops in such a manner so that it is visible to the consumers. Mostly illiterate. Consequently, they do not have any knowledge of microbial contamination which comes after the passage of all the fast moving vehicles on road. While planing this project we thought that the sweets displayed in open pan will have a higher microbial count as compared to sweets displayed in show cases. Therefore, samples of sweets from show cases as well as from open pan were taken for analysis the results so obtained are presented in Tables 3.9 and 3.10.

On the comparison of Tables 3.9 and 3.10 we find that all the average values of standard plate count, spore count and pathogenic count are higher in samples of sweets collected from open pan. It is also clear from the comparison that the difference in average values in all the three tests (S.P.C., Spore and Pathogenic) are more in *peda*. The difference of average pathogenic counts in show cases samples and open pan samples is not significant in *burfi* samples while it is highly significant in *peda* samples. Therefore, we can say if *peda* are sold by keeping them in open pan then the consumers are liable to be effected by Staphylococcal organisms, so as such, they may suffer from gastroenteritis.

Hence, on the comparison of Tables 3.9 and 3.10 we can say that sweets should always kept in show cases. Now-a-days refrigerated show cases are available and they are very good for keeping sweets in good hygienic conditions. Fortunately it is seen that lodge is always kept in show cases. Therefore, except one sample all the samples of lodge have a very low counts.

Summary

To preserve nutritional qualities of milk, it is partially dehydrated into *khoa*. *Khoa* is hardly used as such. However, mixed with sugar and sweets like *burfi*, *peda*, lodge kalakand, etc. are manufactured. The conditions under which these sweets are sold in the market are not always hygienic and so sometimes

Table 3.9

The Result of Microbiological tests applied on sample of burfi, peda and lodge kept in show cases

Sample No.	Burfi			Peda			Lodge		
	S.P.C (10^4)	S.C (10^3)	Pathogens (10^2)	S.P.C (10^4)	S.C (10^3)	Pathogens (10^2)	S.P.C (10^4)	S.C (10^3)	Pathogens (10^2)
1	3.0	7.0	5.0	5.0	8.0	4.0	4.0	29.0	13.0
2	4.0	15.5	5.5	7.5	15.0	6.0	21.0	43.0	17.0
3	—	—	—	—	—	—	6.0	21.5	11.0
4	2.0	32.5	4.0	2.0	30.5	4.5	6.0	6.0	28.0
5	3.5	20.0	4.5	17.5	13.5	15.0	12.0	4.0	2.0
6	11.0	30.0	6.5	23.0	26.0	18.0	7.5	39.0	15.5
7	—	—	—	—	—	—	18.0	44.0	40.0
8	5.5	12.0	9.0	4.0	14.0	—	15.5	66.0	—
9	16.0	28.5	9.5	17.0	16.0	3.0	23.5	77.0	5.5
10	20.5	34.0	7.5	24.0	37.0	2.5	21.5	44.0	9.0
Minimum	2.0	7.0	4.0	2.0	8.0	2.5	4.0	4.0	2.0
Maximum	20.5	34.0	9.5	24.0	37.0	18.0	23.5	77.0	40.0
Average	8.2	22.4	6.4	12.5	20.0	7.6	13.5	37.3	15.7
S. D.	6.447	9.557	2.507	8.310	9.548	5.433	6.967	22.292	11.0

high degree of contamination is expected in these sweets. Therefore, to know the extent of contamination in these sweets this project was taken. In all thirty samples (10 each of *burfi*, *peda* and lodge) were taken from local market. Eight sample were taken from the *halwai* shops selling their sweets from show cases. While only two samples were procured from *halwai* shops selling sweets kept in open pan. But every sample was immediately transferred to laboratory and analysed for the following tests:

A. *Chemical Tests*

1. Moisture percentage
2. Fat percentage
3. Ash percentage
4. Sugar percentage
5. Protein percentage

B. *Microbiological Tests*

1. Standard Plate Count
2. Spore Count
3. Coliform Count
4. Yeast and Mould Count
5. Pathogenic Count

Table 3.10

Sl. No.	Sample No.	Burfi			Peda		
		S.P.C (10^4)	S.C. (10^3)	Pathogen (10^2)	S.P.C (10^4)	S.C. (10^3)	Pathogens (10^2)
1.	3	13.5	41.5	10.5	31.5	11.5	15.0
2.	7	8.0	13.0	3.0	39.5	62.0	35.0
Average		10.7	27.2	6.7	35.5	86.7	25.0

The results of these tests have been presented in Tables 3.1 to 3.8. Standard deviation in every test was also calculated and written in the lower most line of the table.

Moisture percentage in the product definitely affects the shelf life of the product and also its body texture. It is also sometimes adjusted to earn more profit. Consequently, sometimes Government fixes the maximum percentage of moisture in food products. It is clear from Table 3.1 that *burfi* samples have the maximum average moisture percentage (11.83) out of three products. *Burfi* samples also give the lowest range of values (8.10 to 14.30). Next comes *peda* and lastly lodge which has the highest percentage of moisture. The S.D. value of lodge is lowest (1.62). This indicates the uniformity in its day to the production resulting in uniform chemical composition.

For better body and texture, energy and flavour and taste fat percentage in the sweet plays an important role. Therefore, every sample of sweet was analysed for fat percentage by a gravimetric method (Rose Gattlieb). The results so obtained were presented in Table 3.2 after statistical treatment. The lowest average fat percentage (17.90) is reported in *burfi*. It also has the minimum range of values (14.00 to 21.20), having S.D. value 2.08. The highest average fat percentage (26.25) is reported for lodge. Lodge has the highest range also (19.20 to 34.0), having S. D. value 4.91. The *peda* samples give average value and range intermediate to *burfi* and lodge. Therefore, we can place lodge, *peda* and *burfi* in the descending order on the fat content and nutritionally as well, they will be graded in the same order.

Amount of ash indirectly indicates the amount of *khoa* used in the preparation of the sweet. Because when sugar is burnt, it gives no ash. The amount of ash in sweet indicates its mineral richness as well as its nutritional quality. Hence this test was also included in this study and the results have been presented in Table 3.3. It is clear from this table that the highest average ash percentage (2.9) is reported in *peda*, and it has a highest range (1.2-4.8) as well, having S.D. value 1.26. While lodge has got the minimum average ash percentage (2.2) and ash range (1.5 – 3.8) also. The S.D. value is 0.802 only. The average value and range of ash percentage of *burfi* comes in between *peda* and lodge (see Table 3.9). Therefore, we can place lodge, *burfi* and *peda* in an ascending order on the basis of ash percentage.

In order to improve the palatability of sweets sugar is added to *khoa*. It also act as preservative to *khoa*. Sometime sugar is added to earn more profit out of the sweets sale. Therefore, this test was also included in this investigation. The results so obtained have been presented in Table 3.4. It is clear from the table that lodge samples have the average minimum percentage (27.45) and minimum range (22.51-35.95) as well, having S.D. value 4.18. The maximum average sugar percentage is reported for *burfi* (45.47), but the range is not highest. The highest range is seen in *peda* (26.84-54.91), although the average sugar percentage of *peda* lies in between lodge and *burfi*. Therefore, on the basis of sugar percentage lodge, *peda* and *burfi* are placed in an ascending order.

Protein not only important in diet but it is essential in diet, as it provides the amino acids to the consumer. Milk proteins are more important in foods as these protein provides all essential amino acid to the human diet. Therefore, milk proteins are termed as complete proteins. So protein was also determined in sweets, although by difference only. The results are presented in Table 3.5.

It is clear from this table that lodge has got the highest average percentage (28.42) of proteins and the lowest variation in percentages (20.02-37.65) as compared to *peda* (4.29-32.19). But the range is minimum in *burfi* samples (9.88-37.12). Therefore, on the basis of proteins lodge is best, having the highest percentage of proteins, and *peda* the worst, because it has the minimum percentage, *Burfi* comes in between lodge and *peda*.

Standard plate count gives the number of living organisms in any food material. Hence, this test is very widely used in microbiological laboratories. This test was also applied in this investigation and the results, so obtained are presented in Table 3.6. On the perusal of Table 3.6 it is clear that *burfi* samples gave the lowest S.P.C (8.7×10^4/g). The S.D. value was also lowest 5.984, while the *peda* samples gave the highest value (17.1×10^4/g) and the highest variation as well (2.0-39.5×10^4/g). This highest count is due to the vary poor quality of samples no. 3 and 7. Which are actually taken from *halwai* shops where they are kept in open pan. S.P.C. of lodge samples comes in between *burfi* and *peda*. So, on the basis of S.P.C. we can plate *burfi*, lodge and *peda* in ascending order.

Sporing organisms are capable of surviving high temperatures. Therefore, when *khoa* is heated with *bura* only spore bearing organisms survive. It the number of spores is more in any of the *khoa* based sweets then we either suspect poor

Table 3.11

The Average values and range of values of chemical tests applied on samples of Burfi, Peda and Lodge

Constituents	Burfi			Peda			Lodge		
	Minimum	Maximum	Average	Minimum	Maximum	Average	Minimum	Maximum	Average
1. Moisture Percentage	8.10	14.30	11.83 (1.90) ±	10.75	17.10	13.56 (2.14) ±	11.80	17.10	14.72 (1.62) ±
2. Fat Percentage	14.00	21.20	17.90 (2.08) ±	18.20	28.10	23.72 (3.33) ±	19.20	34.00	26.25 (4.91) ±
3. Ash Percentage	1.2	4.5	2.6 (1.06) ±	1.2	4.8	2.9 (1.26) ±	1.5	3.8	2.2 (0.802) ±
4. Sugar Percentage	32.68	58.52	45.47 (8.30) ±	26.84	54.91	39.51 (9.53) ±	22.51	35.98	27.45 (4.18) ±
(Boora)	(36.31)	(65.02)	(50.51) (9.23) ±	(29.81)	(61.00)	(43.90) (10.59) ±	(25.00)	(39.98)	(30.50) (8.86) ±
5. Protein Percentage	9.88	37.12	22.88 (4.84) ±	4.29	32.19	20.25 (7.66) ±	20.02	37.65	28.42 (6.96) ±

Table3.12

The Average values and range of values of Microbiological tests applied on samples of Burfi, Peda and Lodg

Microbiological Tests	Burfi			Peda			Lodge		
	Minimum	Maximum	Average	Minimum	Maximum	Average	Minimum	Maximum	Average
1. Standard Plate Count (×10^4)	2.0	20.5	8.7 (5.984) ±	2.0	39.5	17.1 (11.962) ±	4.0	23.5	13.5 (6.967) ±
2. Spore Count (×10^3)	7.0	41.5	23.4 (10.834) ±	8.0	111.5	33.3 (30.129) ±	4.0	77.0	37.3 (22.292) ±
3. Coliform (×10^2)	—	—	— ±	Only one sample is positive (1×10^2) ±			—	—	— ±
4. Yeast & Mould (×10^2)	—	—	— ±	Only one sample is positive (3×10^2) ±			—	—	— ±
5. Pathogens (×10^2)	3.0	10.5	6.5 (1.483) ±	2.5	35.0	11.4 (10.097) ±	2.0	40.0	15.7 (11.103) ±

quality of *khoa* or *bura* used in the preparation or the heat treatment given was not sufficient. Hence, this count was also included and the results were presented in Tables 3.7 and 3.8 after statistical treatment. It is clear from the table that *burfi* samples are having the lowest average spore count (23.4 × 10³/ g). If *burfi* range is also lowest (7.0-41.5 × 10³/g). Lodge samples give the highest average spore count (37.3 × 10³/g), but the highest range is reported in *peda* (6.0-11.5 × 10³/g). Therefore, on the basis of spore count the we place *burfi*, *peda* and lodge in ascending order.

Coliform, yeasts and moulds they always come from external sources and as such indicated the hygienic conditions prevailing after production of *khoa* based products. Fortunately, all the samples of *burfi* and lodge were free form coliform, yeasts and moulds. However, only one sample of *peda* (sample No. 9) gives the positives coliform test and yeast and mould count, while remaining nine samples are free from these organisms. Therefore, we can say that the hygienic conditions prevailing around the shops are of good condition which have not caused contamination of samples. One thing I would like to write that out of ten eight samples of each product, under study, we procured from sweets kept in show cases which definitely resist the atmospheric contamination.

Therefore, this count was also included in this investigation and results so obtained were tabulated in Table 3.8. This table clearly shows the minimum average pathogenic count (6.5 × 10²/ g) in *burfi* samples. They also give the minimum range (3.0-10.5 × 10²/g), while the average pathogenic count is highest in lodge (15.7 × 10²/g) and the samples are having the maximum variation (2.0-40.0 × 10²/g) too. In *peda* the pathogenic count is in between lodge and *burfi*. On the basis of pathogenic count *burfi* is adjusted the safest, having the minimum pathogenic count, while the highest pathogenic count is reported in lodge and *peda* comes in between.

The average values and range of values for different tests (chemical as well as microbiological) have been presented in summary tables.

Therefore, in the end it can be concluded that on the basis of chemical composition lodge is best nutritionally, as it has highest fat and protein percentages. Next comes *burfi*, because it has the second highest percentage of proteins and last comes *peda*. But microbiologically lodge is worst in quality and due to high moisture and low sugar percentages it can not resist the growth of micro-organisms. Therefore, it is likely to be spoiled quickly. On the other hand microbiologically *burfi* is the best, as its S.P.C., spore count and pathogenic count are lowest. *Peda* comes in between *burfi* and lodge on the basis of all the three tests. Hence, chemically lodge is placed first, *burfi* second and *peda* third, while microbiologically *burfi* placed first, *peda* second and lodge third.

4

DAIRY MICROBIOLOGY

Many organisms can cause mastitis, the most important being *Staphyloccus ourevs, E. coli, Streptoccus alalactiae, S. uberis, Pseudomanas aeruginous* and *Corynebacterium pyogenes*. The first three of these are all potential human pathogens and a number of other human pathogens such as *Salmonella, Listeria moncytogenes, Mycobacterium bovis* and *M. tuberculosis* are also occasionally reported.

1. Cultures

The following standard cultures manufactured in the culture collection of the Dairy Microbiology Division were used in the present study :

- (a) *Streptococcus thermophilus* (HST)
- (b) *Streptococcus thermophilus* (197)
- (c) *Lactobacillus bulgaricus* (Yb)
- (d) *Lactobacillus bulgaricus* (RTS)

The cultures were routinely propagated by overnight transfers in autoclaved (121°C for 15 min.) 100% (w/v) skim milk at their optimum temp. (5-8°C) between semimonthly transfers.

2. Milk Samples

Fresh cow and buffalo ilk samples were collected from cattle yard and Experimental Dai , N.D.R.I., Karnal. Samples were steam sterilized for 30 minutes. Skim milk was obtained by separation of cow milk and sterilized by steaming on 3 successive days.

3. *Media*

For growth studies, the following media were used for :-

(1) *Yeast Dextrose Milk*

Dextrose (D-Glucose)	10 g
Yeast Extract	3 g
Milk	1000 ml.

Sterilized 15 lbs for 25 minutes at 121°C.

(2) *Yeast Dextrose Agar*

Peptone	5 g
Yeast Extract	5 g
Glucose	10 g
Sodium acetate	10 g
Agar	15 g
Distilled water	1000 ml
pH	6.9

(3) *Lactic Agar*

Tryptone	20.0 g
Yeast Extract	5.0 g
Dextrose	5.0 g
Gelatin	2.5 g
Lactose	5.0 g
Sucrose	5.0 g
Sodium Chloride	4.0 g
Sodium Acetate	1.5 g
Ascorbic acid	0.5 g
Distilled water	1000 ml
Agar	15.0 g
pH	6.8 – 7.0

(Before sterilization)

(4) *Trypton Dextrose Agar*

Tryptone	5.0 g

Yeast Extract	2.5 g
D. Glucose	1.0 g
Agar	15.0 g
Distilled water	1000 ml
PH	7.0

(5) Glasswares

All items of glassware used in the study, were cleaned thoroughly using a detergent, dried out and then sterilized in a hot air oven at 160° for 2 hours.

(6) Screening of Culture Combination on the Basis of Acid Production

In both types of milk, the possible culture combination of *Str. thermophilus* and *L. bulgaricus* were evaluated on the basis of total acid production at various periods of incubation.

(7) Chemical Methods For Evaluation of Cultures

Pure and mixed strains cultures of *Str. thermophilus* (Hst) and *L. bulgaricus* (RTS) were inoculated with 16-18 hr old cultures (*L. inoculum*) comprising about 10^7 colony forming units in cow and buffalo milk. The culture ratio was maintained at 1:1 ratio in mixed cultures. Acid production, proteolytic activity, acetaldehyde content and growth were determined using Scientronic pH meter.

(a) *pH* : pH was determined using Scientronic pH meter.
(b) *Tritratable acidity:* Tritratable acidity was measured as percent lactic acid by titrationg a known aliquot of sample 0.1 N NaOH using phenolphthalein as indicator which was added at the rate of 0.5 ml per 10 ml of the sample (Indian Standards Institution, 1960).
(c) *Volatile Acidity* : The volatile acidity was determined (volatile fatty acid) by the method of Hempenius and Liska (1968) with slight modifications.
   Fifty grams of the sample was weighed and transferred to a 1000 ml specially fabricated two necked flask. 3 ml of 1 N H_2SO_4 was added so as to bring down pH to less than

1.0. The contents were then steam distilled and the first 100 ml fraction of the distillate was collected and titrated against 0.1 N NaOH using phenolphthalein indicator and the volatile fatty acids content was expressed as ml of 0.01 N NaOH per 50 g of the sample.

(d) *Proteolytic activity*: Tyrosine value (Hulls' method) was determined by the Hull's with slight modifications.

Reagents

(A) *Trichloracetic acid (TCA)*: 0.72 NTCA solution was prepared by dissolving 58.82 g of TCA in distilled water and the volume was made up to 500 ml (pH 1-2).

(B) Na_2CO_3 *Reagent*: 75 grams of Na_2CO_3 (anhydrous) and 10 g of sodium tri (poly) phosphate were dissolved in distilled water and the volume was made up to 500 ml. pH (above 10.5).

(C) *Folin's Phenol Reagent*: 2N solution and was diluted to 1:1 with distilled water before use.

Procedure

Five grams of the Yoghurt sample and 1 ml distilled water was mixed with 10 ml of 0.72 NTCA solution and incubated at 37°C for 10 min in a thermostatically controlled water bath. The precipitated proteins were filtered through whatman filter paper No. 1 and the tyrosine content in the filterate was determined colorimetrically.

To 0.5 ml of the TCA soluble filterate, 4.5 ml of distilled water was added to make the volume to 5 ml. To this 10 ml of the Na_2CO_3 reagent followed by 3.0 ml of the Folin's phenol reagent (1 N) was added. Mixed well and incubated at 37°C for 5 min for colour development. The intensity of blue colour developed was measured at 660 ml in a Spectrophotometer.

The tyrosine value of the sample was read from a standard curve obtained by treating 5 ml aliquots of the tyrosine solution containing 10-100 µg as described above. The result were expressed as ug of tyrosine per 0.5 ml of TCA filterate.

(e) Acetaldehyde

Reagents

(1) 0.4 g of 3 Methyl-2 bonzothlozolene hydrozeno; hydrochloride in 100 ml of distilled water.
(2) Dimethyl sulfoxide, APR.
(3) 0.2 g of $FeCl_3$ (A.R.) in 100 ml 0.1 N HCl.
(4) Acetone A. R.

Procedure

Ten grams of sample was weighed and made up to 20 g with distilled water in a sample test tube. The sample was added with a little amount of antifoaming agent and the test tube was fitted with a collection trap which contained 2.5 ml of distilled water, 2.5 ml of 0.4% MBTH and 0.5 ml of Dimethyl Sulphoxide. The collection system was assembled and the tube with the culture were placed in a water bath at 65°C and purged with 100-125 ml of nitrogen gas per minute for 1 hour.

The trap was then disconnected and the initial reaction was allowed to proceed to completion by holding the trap at room temperature for 25 min. 12.5 ml of 0.2% $FeCl_3$ in 0.1 N HCl was then added and the mixture was allowed to stand exactly for 25 min at which time 20 ml of acetone was added and mixed immediately to stop the oxidation reaction. The contents of the reaction mixture was then transferred to a 55 ml volumetric flask and the volume was made up with acetone. The absorbance at 660 nm was determined within 30 min by reading against a similarly handled reagent blank with a Pye Unicham Spectrophotometer.

Preparation of Standard Curve

A standard curve was prepared by adding dilutions of acetaldehyde directly to the collection reagent, followed by the regular procedure for colour development.

The acetaldehyde content in the sample can be directly read on the standard curve corresponding to the absorbance at 660 nm.

```
┌──────────────────┐          ┌──────────────────┐
│ Fruit/Sweetened  │          │ Plain Yoghurt ˙  │
│    Yoghurt       │          └──────────────────┘
└──────────────────┘                   │
         │                  ┌──────────────────┐      ┌──────────────────┐
         │                  │ Milk (cow/buffalo)│─────│ (Perform compo-  │
         │                  └──────────────────┘      │   sitional test  │
         │                           │                └──────────────────┘
         │                  ┌──────────────────┐         (A) Adjust fat (2-3%)
         │                  │ Standardisation  │         (B) Add SMP (2%)
         │                  └──────────────────┘         (C) Add gelatin (0.5%)
         │                        Stir
         │                  ┌──────────────────┐
         │                  │ Homogenisation   │
         │                  └──────────────────┘
         │                           │
         │                  ┌──────────────────┐      ┌──────────────────┐
         │                  │ Heat treatment   │─────│ (Steaming for    │
         │                  └──────────────────┘      │  30 minutes)     │
         │                        Stir                └──────────────────┘
┌──────────────────┐       ┌──────────────────┐      ┌──────────────────┐
│ Add sugar (5-6%) │       │ Inoculation with │─────│ S. thermophilus +│
└──────────────────┘       │ yoghurt starter (3%)     │  L. bulgarlcus  │
         │                 └──────────────────┘      └──────────────────┘
         │                        Stir
┌──────────────────┐
│ Add fruit pulp   │
│   (15-20%)       │
└──────────────────┘
    Stir                   ┌──────────────────┐      ┌──────────────────┐
         │                 │   Incubation     │      │ Subjective tests │
         └─────────────────│ (45°C for 3.5 hours)    │ (Sensory evaluation)
                           └──────────────────┘      │  A. Body         │
                                   │                 │  B. Texture      │
                                   │                 │  C. Flavour      │
                                   │                 └──────────────────┘
                           ┌──────────────────┐      ┌──────────────────┐
                           │ Cooling (20°C)   │      │ Objective tests  │
                           │ and quality      │      │ (Laboratiry      │
                           │ evaluation       │      │   analysis       │
                           └──────────────────┘      │  A. Chemical     │
                                   │                 │  B. Physical     │
                           ┌──────────────────┐      │  C. Microbiology │
                           │ Storage at 5°c   │      └──────────────────┘
                           └──────────────────┘
```

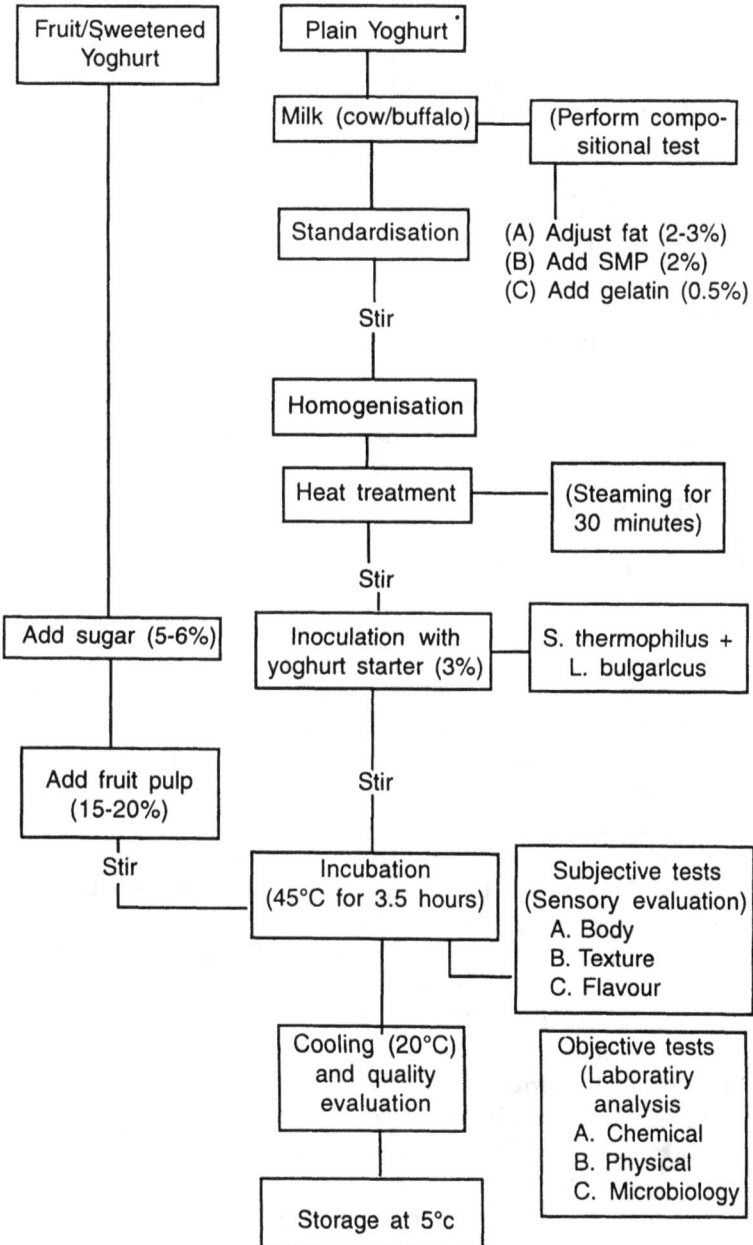

Procedure for the Manufacture and Quality Evaluation of Plain/
Sweetened/Fruit Yoghurt

(8) Preparation of Yoghurt

Three types of yoghurt, namely, plain yoghurt, fruit yoghurt and sweetened yoghurt were prepared by the procedure indicated in the flow sheet. A conventional method for the preparation of yoghurt is as below:

Cow and buffalo milk samples were steamed for 30 min, cooled to a temp. of 43°C and then inoculated at 3% level with 16-18 hrs old cultures of *Str. thermophilus* and *L. bulgaricus* in equal proportions (1 : 1).

The cotnents were mixed thoroughly and filled into 250 ml glass bottles, covered with the lids or aluminium foil caps, were transferred to a water bath maintained at 42°C ± 0.5°C. After incubation for 2.5-3.0 hrs when the coagulum was formed the bottles were then removed from the water bath, cooled at 30° for ½ hr and then transferred to refrigeration for overnight storage.

Result and Discussion

Different culture combination of *Str. thermophilus* (HST, 197) and *Lactobacillus bulgaricus* (RTS, Yb) for total acid production in cow milk (Table 4.1) and buffalo milk (Table 4.2) from 2-10 hrs of incubation. It is evident that with increase in incubation time there was an increase in acid production in the culture combinations of different strains in both the types of milk. Earlier reports by Calesloot (1960), Mocquot and Hurrel (1970) and Tramer (1973) have indicated that selection of different strains of lactic cultures depends on the availability of the organism to grow together in order to attain the desirable acid production. It was interesting to note that mixed cultures of *Str. thermophilus* (HST) + *L. bulgaricus* (RTS), *Str. thermophilus* (197) + *L. bulgaricus* (Yb) and *Str. thermophilus* (197) + *L. bulgaricus* (RTS), *Str. thermophilus* (HST) + *L. bulgaricus* (Yb) exhibited more and production after 10 hrs of incubation, irrespective of the type of milk used. It was found that acid production by above mixed cultures varied from 1.02 – 1.10% and 1.05-1.22% lactic acid in cow and buffalo milk respectively. Based on uniform and greater acid production the mixed culture of *Str. thermophilus* (HST) and *L. bulgaricus* (RTS) was selected for further study.

Effect of different incubation periods on developed acidity. pH Volatile acidity, proteolytic activity and acetaldehyde production by *Str. thermophilus* (HST) and *L. bulgaricus* (RTS) in cow and buffalo milk, have been mentioned in Tables 4.3-4.10.

Table 4.1
Total acid production by different combinations fo *L. bulgaricus* and *Str. thermophilus* in cow milk

Sr. No.	Culture	Titratable Acidity % Lactic Acid				
		2 hr	4 hr	6 hr	8 hr	10 hr
1.	*L. bulgaricus* (RTS) + *Str. Thermophilus* (Hst)	0.31	0.44	0.72	0.90	1.09
2.	*L. bulgaricus* (Yb) + *Str. thermophilus* (197)	0.36	0.46	0.77	0.94	1.06
3.	*L. Bulgaricus* (Yb) + *Str. thermophilus* (HST)	0.32	0.48	0.66	0.90	0.93
4.	*L. bulgaricus* (RTS) + *Str. thermophilus* (197)	0.28	0.44	0.81	0.94	1.03

Table 4.2
Total Acid Production by different combinations fo *L. bulgaricus* and *Str. thermophilus* in buffalo milk

Sr. No.	Culture	Titratable Acidity % Lactic Acid				
		2 hr	4 hr	6 hr	8 hr	10 hr
1.	*L. bulgaricus* (RTS) + *Str. Thermophilus* (Hst)	0.34	0.56	0.89	1.10	1.26
2.	*L. bulgaricus* (Yb) + *Str. thermophilus* (197)	0.31	0.51	0.82	0.91	0.99
3.	*L. Bulgaricus* (Yb) + *Str. thermophilus* (HST)	0.37	0.56	0.71	0.88	0.98
4.	*L. bulgaricus* (RTS) +I *Str. thermophilus* (197)	0.39	0.46	0.86	0.96	1.07

A. Acid Production

From the results in Tables 4.3-4.4, it is evident that there was a progressive increase in the developed acidity (Table 4.3 and 4.4) and decrease in pH value (Tables 4.5 and 4.6) of pure and mixed culture of *Str. thermophilus* and *L. bulgaricus* (RTS) with increase in incubation period irrespective of the type of milk used. Pure culture of above organism shoed less developed acidity in both the types of milk as compared to their mixture udder similar experimental conditions. These results are in accordance with the findings of Potte and Lolkema (1950), Rabranzlev (1954), Ashlon (1963) and Accolan *et al.* (1977) who obtained rapid and higher acid production in mixed cultures of *Str. thermophilus* and *L. bulgaricus* in milk than the corresponding single strain.

Table 4.3
Effect of different incubation periods on the developed acidity of pure and mixed strain cultures of *Str. Thermophilus* and *L. bulgaricus* in cow milk

Sr. No.	Culture	% developed acidity				
		2 hr	6 hr	10 hr	14 hr	18 hr
1.	*L. bulgaricus* (RTS)	0.05	0.13	0.25	0.61	0.73
2.	*Str. thermophahilus* (HST)	0.04	0.31	0.54	0.60	0.62
3.	Expected value (sum of the developed acidity of the both cultures)	0.09	0.44	0.79	1.21	1.35
4.	*L. bulgaricus* (RTS) *Str. thermophilus* (HST)	0.14	0.65	0.90	0.92	0.94

Each value is average of two trails in duplicate.

Stimulation of acid production in mixed culture of 0.5% *Str. thermophilus* (HST) and 0.5% *L. bulgaricus* (RTS) was studied and it was observed that for the first 11 hrs and 9 hrs of incubation in cow and buffalo milk respectively (Table 4.3 and 4.4), the stimulation of the mixed culture was evident. These results are in conformity with earlier reports by moon and Reinbold (1978) who observed increased developed acidity for first 10 hrs of incubation in skim milk, pure and mixed cultures developed more acidity and less pH in buffalo milk than cow milk. Thomas *et al.* (1966) showed that rate of acid production by lactic cultures was higher in buffalo milk than in cow milk. Considerable variations in acid production y lactic cultures grown in milk of different species was observed by Dutta *et al.* (1971) and Singh and Ranganathan (1978).

Table 4.4
Effect of different incubation periods on the developed acidity
pure and mixed strain cultures of *Str. Thermophilus* and
***L. bulgaricus* in buffalo milk**

Sr. No.	Culture	% developed acidity				
		2 hr	6 hr	10 hr	14 hr	18 hr
1.	*L. bulgaricus* (RTS)	0.05	0.14	0.38	0.67	0.81
2.	*Str. thermophahilus* (HST)	0.07	0.37	0.56	0.62	0.68
3.	Expected value (sum of the developed acidity of the both cultures)	0.12	0.51	0.94	1.29	1.49
4.	*L. bulgaricus* (RTS) *Str. thermophilus* (HST)	0.26	0.80	0.98	1.07	1.14

Each value is average of two trails in duplicate.

B. Proteolytic Activity

Data in Tables 4.9 and 4.10 relate to effect of periods of incubation on proteolytic activity of pure and mixed cultures of *Str. thermophilus* and *L. bulgaricus* in cow and buffalo mill. Proteolytic activity of pure and mixed cultures of both types of milk increases with increase in incubation time.

However, *L. bulgaricus* exhibit more proteolytic activity (0.53 and 0.62 mg tyrosine/g of curd) than *Str. thermophilus* (0.30 and 0.36 mg tyrosine/g of curd) in cow and buffalo milk respectively after 24 hours. These results are in confirmation with earlier reports of Searles *et al.* (1970), Nachev (1969) and Dutta *et al.* (1970) who recorded that lactobacilli possessed greater proleolytic activity as compared to streptococci.

Pure and mixed cultures of *Str. thermophilus* showed more proteolytic activity in buffalo than in cow milk (Tables 4.9 and 4.10). These results are in contradiction to the results presented by

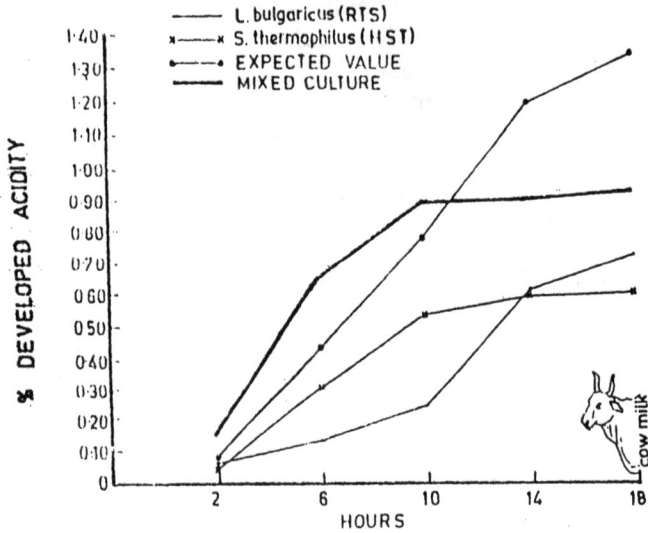

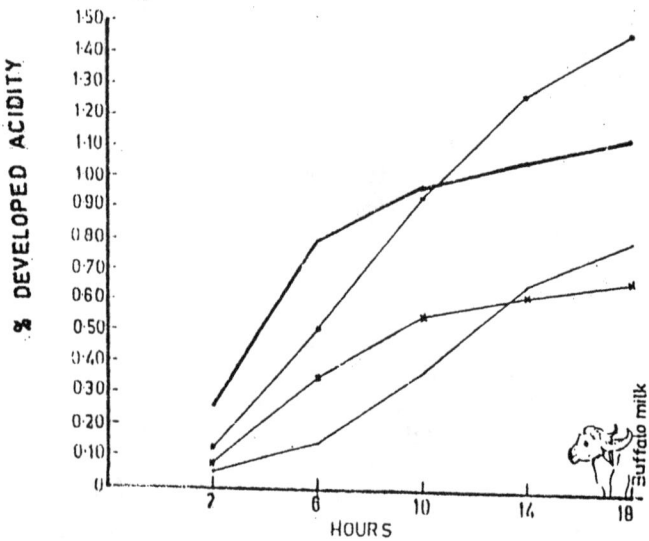

Fig. 4.1: Percentage Acidity of Mixed and Pure Cultures of Cow's and buffalo's Milk

Table 4.5

Effect of different incubation periods of pH of pure and mixed strain cultures of Streptococcus thermophillus and Lactobacillus bulgaricus in cow milk.

Sr. No.	Culture	pH									
		0 hr	3 hr	6 hr	9 hr	12 hr	15 hr	18 hr	21 hr	24 hr
1.	Control	6.70	6.70	6.65	6.62	6.60	6.60	6.60	6.57	6.52
2.	*L. bulgaricus* (RTS)	6.55	6.30	6.00	5.35	4.60	4.40	4.30	4.05	3.75
3.	*Str. thermophilus* (Hst)	6.60	5.95	5.80	5.60	4.80	4.60	4.40	4.35	4.30
4.	*L. bulgaricus* (RTS) + *Str. thermophilus* (Hst)	6.60	5.45	5.30	4.95	4.55	4.50	4.20	3.90	3.60

Each value is a mean of two trails in duplicate.

Table 4.6

Effect of different incubation periods of pH of pure and mixed strain cultures of Streptococcus thermophillus and Lactobacillus bulgaricus in buffalo milk.

Sr. No.	Culture	pH								
		0 hr	3 hr	6 hr	9 hr	12 hr	15 hr	18 hr	21 hr	24 hr
1.	Control	6.70	6.70	6.65	6.62	6.60	6.60	6.60	6.57	6.52
2.	L. bulgaricus (RTS)	6.55	6.15	6.00	5.90	4.50	4.30	3.80	3.70	3.40
3.	Str. thermophilus (Hst)	6.55	6.00	5.70	5.65	4.70	4.20	4.10	4.15	4.00
4.	L. bulgaricus (RTS) + Str. thermophilus (Hst)	6.55	6.10	5.60	5.00	4.60	4.30	3.70	3.50	3.40

Each value is a mean of two trails in duplicate.

Thomas *et al.* (1966). Mixed cultures of *Str. thermophilus* and *L. bulgaricus* showed decrease in proteolytic activity as compared to pre cultures of *L. bulgaricus*. For instance mixed cultures showed 0.36 and 0.40 mg tyrone, while L. *bulgaricus* liberated (0.53 and 0.62 mg tyrone in cow and buffalo milk. These results are in agreement to Formisano *et al.* (1970) who noted similar variations in the proteolytic activity of mixed cultures of *Str. thermophilus* and *L. bulgaricus*.

Table 4.7
Volatile acid production by pure and mixed strain cultures of *Streptococcus thermophilus* and *Lactobacillus bulgaricus* at different hours of incubation in cow milk

Sl. No.	Culture	Volatile acidity (ml. 0.IN NaOH used/50 g of curd)				
		4 hrs	8 hrs	12 hrs	16 hrs	20 hrs
1.	L. *bulgaricus* (RTS)	1.00	3.10	4.40	4.80	4.90
2.	*Str. thermophilus* (Hst)	0.64	1.20	1.70	2.00	2.30
3.	L. *bulcaricus* (RTS) *Str. thermophilus* (Hst)	3.00	5.10	6.90	7.50	7.80

Each trail is a mean of two trials in duplicate

Table.4.8
Volatile acid production by pure and mixed strain cultures of *Streptococcus thermophilus* and *Lactobacillus bulgaricus* at different hours of incubation in buffalo milk

Sl. No.	Culture	Volatile acidity (ml. 0.IN NaOH used/50 g of curd)				
		4 hrs	8 hrs	12 hrs	16 hrs	20 hrs
1.	L. *bulgaricus* (RTS)	1.70	4.00	5.30	6.20	7.00
2.	*Str. thermophilus* (Hst)	0.50	1.60	2.30	2.60	2.70
3.	L. *bulcaricus* (RTS) *Str. thermophilus* (Hst)	1.40	6.00	7.40	8.00	8.50

Each trail is a mean of two trials in duplicate

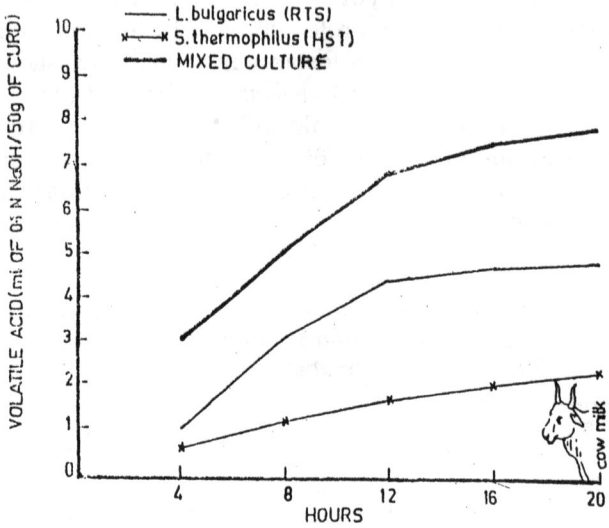

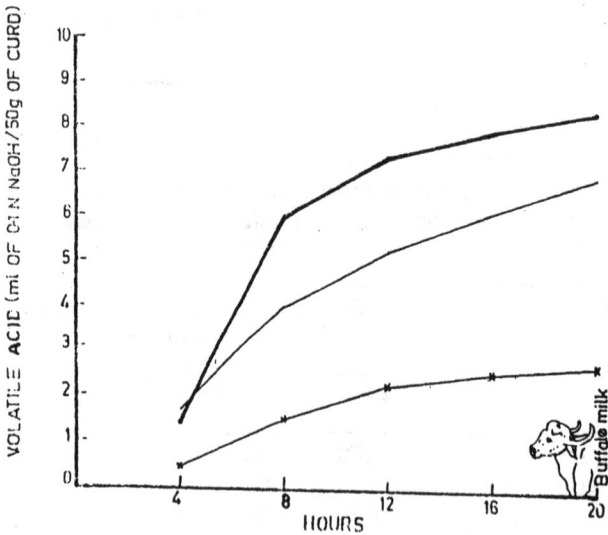

Fig. 4.2: Volatile Acid Production of Mixed and Pure Cultures of
Cow's and buffalo's Milk

Table 4.9

Effect of different incubation period son the proteolytic activity of pure and mixed strain culture of *Str. thermophilus* and *L. bulgaricus* in cow milk

Sl. No.	Culture	mg of Tyrosine liberatred/g of curd									
		0 hrs	3 hrs	6 hrs	9 hrs	12 hrs	15 hrs	18 hrs	21 hrs	24 hrs
1.	*L. bulgaricus* (RTS)	0.08	0.14	0.18	0.27	0.31	0.41	0.46	0.49	0.53
2.	*Str. thermophilus* (Hst)	0.09	0.12	0.15	0.17	0.22	0.24	0.27	0.28	0.30
3.	*L. bulcaricus* (RTS) *Str. thermophiilus* (Hst)	0.09	0.12	0.15	0.23	0.23	0.29	0.31	0.34	0.36

Each trail is a mean of two trials in duplicate

Table 4.10

Effect of different incubation periodds on the proteolytic activity of pure and mixed strain culture of *Str. thermophilus* and *L. bulgaricus* in buffalo milk.

Sl. No.	Culture	mg of Tyrosine liberatred/g of curd								
		0 hrs	3 hrs	6 hrs	9 hrs	12 hrs	15 hrs	18 hrs	21 hrs	24 hrs
1.	*L. bulgaricus* (RTS)	0.09	0.23	0.30	0.36	0.46	0.50	0.56	0.59	0.62
2.	*Str. thermophilus* (Hst)	0.09	0.15	0.21	0.24	0.28	0.29	0.32	0.34	0.36
3.	*L. bulcaricus* (RTS) *Str. thermophilus* (Hst)	0.10	0.16	0.22	0.28	0.30	0.34	0.36	0.38	0.40

Each trail is a mean of two trials in duplicate

C. *Flavour Production*

The delicate and pleasing flavour of yoghurt can be attributed to appreciable amounts of acetaldehyde and volatile acid production by *L. bulgaricus* and *Str. thermophilus*. Results on the effect of different incubation periods on the volatile acid production and acetaldehyde content of pure and mixed cultures of *Str. thermophilus* and *L. bulgaricus* have been recorded in Tables 4.7-4.8. There was an increase in volatile acidity in *Str. thermophilus* and *L. bulgaricus* with the incubation period irrespective of the type of milk used. Variation with regard to volatile acid production was noted in buffalo milk as compared to cow milk after 6 hrs of incubation. However, pure end mixed cultures of *Str. thermophilus* and *L. bulgaricus* exhibited more volatile acid production in buffalo than a cow milk after 4-20 hrs of incubation.

At the initiation of incubation between pure and mixed cultures of *Str. thermophilus* and *L. bulgaricus* which increase after 2 hrs in both types of milk. Mixed cultures produced more acetaldehyde

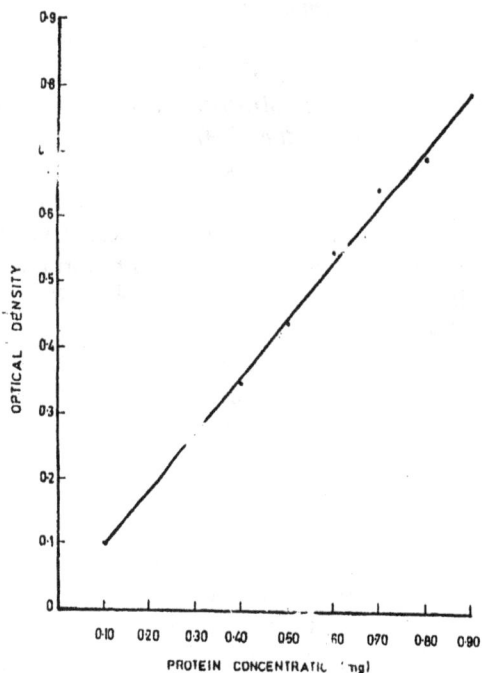

Fig. 4.3: Standrad Curve for Tyro ine Estimation

as compared to *Str. thermophilus* and *L. bulgaricus* at the same hour in cow and buffalo milk. At 12 hr of incubation, *L. bulgaricus* and mixed culture exhibited a decrease I acetaldehyde production, irrespective of the type of milk used. Gorner *et al.* (1968) found that acetaldehyde is the only compound liberated by lactic culture which was responsible for favour of yoghurt. *L. bulgaricus* produce more acetaldehyde than *Str. thermophilus* but still below that fromed by the combined organisms. Similar trend in the acetaldehyde production by pure and mixed cultures of *Str. thermophilus* and *L. bulgaricus* were observed in cow and buffalo milk. These results confirm the symbiotic relationship that exhibit between the two organisms and indicated by Pette and Lolkema (1950) and Bautista *et al.* (1966).

Growth of pure and mixed cultures of Str. thermophilus and L. bulgaricus in cow and buffalo milk

Several workers have studied the symbiotic relationship in mixed cultures of *Str. thermophilus* and *L. bulgaricus* (Pette and Lolakema, 1950; Bautista *et al.* 1966; Galesloot et al., 1968; Accolas *et al.*, 1971 and Higashio *et al.* (1978), there are only a few reports on the associative growth of *Str. thermophilus* and *L. bulgaricus*. Bautista *et al.* (1966). Accolas *et al.* (1971) and Moon and Reinbold (1976) found that greater acid production in mixed culture was due to enhanced growth of streptococci. The results repored in the present study further confirms this point. There was a significant increase in growth of *Str. thermophilus* at 8 hrs in cow milk and 4 hrs in buffalo milk. Later, viable number of *Str. thermophilus* decreased in the mixture and to a less extent in the control irrespective of the milk used. Growth of *L. bulgaricus* in mixed cultures was less vigorous than in control in both the types of milk. These results are in accordance with the finding of Moon and Reinbold (1976) indicating the inhibition of *L. bulgaricus* throughout its incubation in mixed cultures. Inhibition of an organism in mixed culture may be therapeutically due to crowding, pH competition for nutrients of presence of inhibitory compound.

At optimal condition for stimulation of acid production, *Str. thermophilus* grew much more rapidly than *L. bulgaricus*. A competitive growth advantage of *Str. thermophilus* is suggested by the temperature optium for stimulation, 37°C. This temperature to the optimum growth temperature for *Str. thermophilus* (42-45°C) than for *L. bulgaricus* (45-50°C).

Summary

1. Different strains of *Str. thermophilus* and L. *bulgaricus* was evaluated fore total acid production in cow and buffalo milk from 0-10 hrs at 37°C. Based on uniform and greater acid production, the culture combination of *Str. thermophilus* (HST) and L. *bulgaricus* (RTS) were used for further studies.

2. Pure cultures of *Str. thermophilus* and L. *bulgaricus* exhibited less developed acidity in both types of milk as compared to their mixtures.

3. Pure and mixed cultures developed more acidity and less pH in buffalo milk than in cow milk.

4. Pure and mixed cultures of *Str. thermophilus* and L. *bulgaricus* showed increased proteolytic activity with increase in incubation lime.

5. Mixed cultures of *Str. thermophilus* and L. *bulgaricus* showed decreased in proteolytic activity as compared to L. *bulgaricus* in both types of milk.

6. Pure and mixed cultures produced more volatile acid in buffalo milk than in cow milk.

7. Mixed cultures of *Str. thermophilus* and L. *bulgaricus* produced more acetaldehyde as compared to pure culture after 10 hrs of incubation. However, after which L. *bulgaricus* and mixed cultures showed in decrease in acetaldehyde production irrespective of the type of milk.

8. *Str. thermophilus* produced more growth at 8 hrs in cow milk and 4 hrs in buffalo milk. In mixed culture the number of *Str. thermophilus* decreased and to a less extent in the control irrespective of the milk used.

9. Growth of L. *bulgaricus* in mixed culture was less vigorous than in control in both the types of milk.

5

BUTTER MICROBIOLOGY

A. Importance of Butter Manufacture in India

The fat content of butter is generally about 80%. The non-fat components of butter consists of moisture, milk soil not fat and salt.

Conservation of milk of fat in the form of either butter for direct consumption or it's derivative ghee, is one of the most ancient and important methods of utilising milk for manufacture of milk products in India. In western countries the term "butter" always refers to " Creamery butter "which in derived from the churning of cream and is used for table purposes. Another type of butter that is prepared from soured milk or *dahi* in India is called *"desi* butter". The latter product is mainly clarified into ghee and stored over long periods. Butter is made from sweet or sour cream. The cream is pasteurised at 62.8°C for 30 minutes often which is immediately cooled.

Butter is defined as a food product which is made with or without additional colouring matter and contains about 80% (by weight) of milk fat (Prescott and Proctor, 1937). It is a water in fat emulsion in which the continuous phase is semi solid. The emulsion consists of dispersed fat globules, moisture droplets and air, each being stabilised by an envelope of protein material. The chief component of butter is butter-fat which comprises at least 80% of butter. It also contains small amounts of ash, acids, phospholipids and air besides enzymes and vitamins.

The butter constitutes a major branch of dairy industry and is the chief means of conserving the valuable nutritive properties of milk fat in a less perishable form. Many countries of the world not only produce large quantities of butter but also have established a flourishing export trade. In India milk fat is chiefly converted into country or *desi* butter which is subsequently clarified into *ghee*. The marketable value and nutritive properties of butter are however, governed by it's quality, it's physical appearance, texture, flavour and chemical composition. The properties desired in high quality butter are:

1. Sweet fresh and clean flavour
2. Firm and uniform body.
3. Pleasing and light colour which may vary from light straw to yellow.
4. If salted. Salting should be medium and evenly distributed; and
5. Moisture should be at a minimum (16%) and without free water droplets.

In addition, the product should be free from pathogenic organisms in order to be considered fit for human consumption and possess good keeping quality, if it has to with stand prolonged storage or transport over long distance in a satisfactory condition. All these in turn depend on the exact methods of manufacture employed and the extent of care and hygienic standard exercised in the preparation and handling of butter.

B. Methods of Manufacture of Butter In India

(i) Desi

In India the desi method of butter-making is most prevalant, mainly as an intermediate process in *ghee* manufacture. It is only recently that creamery butter manufacture is assuming increasing significance. It is claimed that 97.5% (Chandraban, 1940) of the total ghee produced is made from *desi*-butter and the latter accounts for 86% (Devies, 1939) of the total butter produced in India. Although this method is being practised since a long time, the conditions of it's manufacture at present are generally unsatisfactory.

(ii) Creamery

In general butter manufacturing practice, milk is separated in a centrifugal cream separator, the fat percentage of cream being adjusted to 25 to 33%. It is repened, for 12 to 24 hours by seeding it with 2 to 5% of good butter starter containing a suitable combination of acid and aroma producing organisms. The ripened cream is then churned either on the same day or after collecting the lots of cream for two or three days. After churning, the butter is washed and worked and about 1% of common salt added. The butter is then moulded in woolen dyes and packed in butter paper. The butter paper packets are kept in the refrigerator or in the cold store till they are disposed off. There are, however many variations in actual practice. The quality of milk, or cream collected from different sources, use of unpasteurised and even ùnripened cream, use of unclean butter churn and other equipment, impure water for washing or contaminated wrappers etc., may constitute important factors in the contamination of butter with various types of micro-organisms.

C. Microflora of Butter

(1) Microbial Numbers In Butter

It is evident that the bacterial content of fresh butter is extremely variable depending primarily on the methods of manufacture, as also on temperature, salt content, air supply acidity, physical condition etc. of butter. Thus, in butter made from unpasteurised milk or cream kept at low temperature, water bacteria will tend to predominate, while at ordinary temperature the sweet butter will soon become sour owing to the rapid development of lactic acid streptococci. Later on lactic acid bacteria, yeasts and moulds appear. Butter made form pasteurised ripened milk or cream will have a much simpler flora to begin with, as *Streptococcus cremoris* used in the ripening process will generally be the principle organism present. This organism dies not seem to be capable of living long in butter and is gradually replaced by lactobacilli and then yeasts.

The number of micro-organisms in butter will depend on the nature and amount of nutrient butter and inhibitory substances present in the water droplets, i.e. on the washing, working and addition of salt. Properly handled butter seldom contains more than a few million bacteria per cubic centimeter. In butter from ripened cream, the count is highest when the butter is freshly made and decreases from day to day, the reason being that the original, lactic acid bacteria die off at a quicker rate than their successors develop, since the available nutrient matter, especially lactose. Is continuously decreasing. Similarly the number of yeasts and moulds also vary. Conn (1930) reported about 26,000,000 organisms in a sample of butter one day old, 2,000,000 in 4 days and 300.000 in 30-days old butter.

(2) Sources of Bacterial Contamination in Butter

The methods of manufacture and handling of butter not only determines the composition, body and flavour, but also offer very wide scope for numerous organisms to enter it from various sources, including milk or cream, the butter culture, the equipment, the wash water, the air, the personal and package.

(a) *Cream*: Macy Coulter and Combs (1932) studying 45 lots of cream, found the total bacterial, yeast and mould counts ranging from 1.520,000 to 160,000,000 per ml., 50 to 14,510 per ml., 2 to 32,000 per ml. respectively. In the case of sour cream intended for conversion into butter, hundreds of millions of bacteria per ml, including starter organisms and large numbers of yeasts and moulds may be present. They reported that nearly all the bacteria and 89 to 100% of the yeasts and all the mould were destroyed by pasteurisation. Powell (1938) found acid congulating organisms predominating in fresh cream but during storage they were replaced by acid forming, acid coagulating and peptonizing groups. Deterioration of the quality of cream accompanied by Anderson and Hardenberg (1932) resulting in bitter flavour. Pont (1935) isolated from cream a number of strains of coliform bacteria causing rapid and serious deterioration. Crossley (1939) also found coliform bacteria in clotted cream. Among the variety of fungi which may be originally present in cream, Oidium lactis is probably the best known. According to Elliker (1941) the source of it's contamination in cream are dust, dirt, manure and unclean utensils.

(b) *Starter*: When butter culture is added to the milk or cream, most of the culture organisms are held in the butter milk, but some appear in the finished product (Orla-Jensen, 1931). The organisms appearing in butter depends upon whether the starter is contaminated or not. Vats, coolers, pumps, piping etc., may be sources of contamination and adequate methods of cleaning and sterlisation are necessary.

(c) *Churn*: Churns constitute an important source of micro-organisms. The surface of the wood is more or less irregular. The irregular surface increases as the wood takes up water and the wood may crack so that removal of organisms and milk stone become difficult. Several workers have emphasized the importance of churns as a source of organisms in butter. Thus for example, Macy, Combs and Morrison (1931) by dismantling two churns which were in use for a long time demonstrated that numerous foci of contamination existed in the churns. Olson and Hammer (1934) found that 27 churns in commercial use in 24 plants varied widely n their microbiological condition, some containing small and others excessive numbers. Bacterial numbers were always more numerous in the churns than yeasts or moulds. Stiritz   (1922) observed that the churn may be one of the greatest sources of contamination of cream after pasteurization.

(d) *Wash Water:* Water is a very important source of contamination and frequently in pure water used for washing the butter has led to the lapied deterioration of butter Stiritz (1922) Sorensen (1940), Linneboe (1940), Wolchow, Thronton and Wood (1941). The wash water retained in butter and the water used to adjust the moisture content of butter are probably never as finely distributed as that which was originally present in the cream. The types of organisms derived from water probably affects the keeping quality more than those derived from cream. Therefore an organism from added water is more serious from the stand point of deterioration, provided the other conditions in the butter permits it's growth.

(e) *Air:* Air contamination in butter manufacture is important because butter is often exposed during packing and is frequently held for relatively long periods at temperatures permitting the growth of organisms resulting especially in the development of moulds on butter. Olson and Hammer (1934) studied the numbers of bacteria, yeasts and moulds falling from the air and found that amongst the three bacteria were the most numerous and yeasts the least numerous. The results showed the constant danger of organisms falling in the surface of exposed butter, moulds constituting the most serious contamination from the air. Butter held under conditions permitting the growth of organisms often show higher counts at the surface than in the interior and certain microbiological defects are first evidenced on the surface. This may be interpreted as due to the effect of air supply on the growth of these organisms.

In order to reduce bacterial contamination and control the activity of undesirable organisms, a number of methods have been employed, the most important ones being, pasteurisation (Hunziker, 1940; Fettick, 1908; Thom and Shaw, 1915), addition of preservatives (Elson and Walker, 1942) and low temperature storage (Loftus-Hills *et al.*, 1934). The problem of preserving butter in a good condition still presents exceptional difficulties particularly in a tropical country like India where some of the methods employed for controlling bacterial activities are either not in use or cannot be applied with the same degree of success.

3. Spoilage of Butter

As a result of careless methods, employment of unclean equipment, use of unpasteurised milk or cream, storage at high temperature and other causes, butter may undergo serious changes in it's composition and develop various defects.

(a) *Rancidity:* A flavour suggestive of butyric and caproic acids often develops in butter and is described as rancid. These acids are set free through hydrolysis of fat and are generally due to micro-organisms present in butter. The early work of Orla-Jensen (1902) demonstrated that certain species of micro-organisms such as *Oidium lactis, Cladosporcum butyri, Bacillus prodigious* as also certain lipolytic strains of Pseudomonas and Achromobacter (Hammer and Collins, 1934), are capable of hydrolysing the fat in butter to a market degree and of producing an intensely rancid flavour. Organisms producing rancidity in butter are widely distributed and commonly present in raw cream. They are easily destroyed by pasteurisation so that with adequate protection against contamination there is little chance of this defect appearing.

(b) *Tallowincess:* Like rancidity, tallowy flavour is also due to a decomposition of the fat. However, while rancidity is due to fat hydrolysis, by lipolytic bacteria, tallowiness is caused by the oxidation of fat, involving the unsaturated fatty acids in butter, such as oleic acid. It is a taint which develops in pure fats or fat rich material and is regarded as a state of comparatively advanced stage of oxidation of fat. The defect varies from a very slight abnormality to an extreme condition in which the off-flavour is pronounced and the butter may even be bleached. The development of tallowiness in sterile butter indicates that the direct action of orgainsms is not involved. Hunziker and Hosman (1917) concluded that tallowiness results from the oxidation of butter fat but that the product which is necessary to link up with the fatty acids to make it tallowy is derived from free glycerol produced by hydrolysis of fat. King (1931) noted that in presence of air, butter fat reacted with diacetyl and became tallowy and bleached. The reaction is accelerated by light. He suggested that diacetyl may act on butter fat by oxidising oleic acid to oleic acid peroxide which then breaks up into various compounds having a pronounced tallowy flavour, the diacetyl being reduced to acetyl methyl carbinol.

(c) *Fishiness:* The development of a fishy falvour in butter is one of the most serious types of deterioration. It is primarily a defect of butter that has been stored, but occasionally appears in fresh butter, when the acidity of cream at churning is relatively high. O'Callaghan (1901) cited experiments which suggested that *Oidium lactis* was the cause of the defect. Later O'Callaghan (1907) has reported that when this organism was grown in conjunction with *S. lactis*, fishiness was produced on every occasion.

Rogers (1909) concluded from his study of fishy butter that flavour is evidently not produced by the action of any one special factor. He noted that acid is essential and that butter made from pasteurised sweet cream with a butter, culture, but without ripening, seldom if ever becomes fishy. Klein (1914) speaking of Oily, fishy and tallowy butter, holds that all these defects may be considered specific forms of rancid butter, resulting from the action of bacteria.

However Reakes, Cuddie and Reid (1912) were unable to find significant differences in the bacteria of fishy and high grade butter. Sommer and Smit (1923) pointed out that pasteurisation tends to eliminate fishiness, because it causes some hydrolysis of lecithin, the products of which are lost in butter-milk.

(d) *Surface Taint:* In butter, a defect commonly described as surface taint, has been encountered very often. The defect begins at the surface and at comparatively high temperatures, may develop quite rapidly. According to Hood and White (1928) it is noticed in first-grade pasteurised cream butter. These investigators noted that butter with this defect showed abnormally high yeast and bacterial counts and that all samples contained large numbers of bacteria capable of decomposing the curd.

Derby and Hammer (1931) found that butter having a surface taint often contained large numbers of bacteria although in a few samples the counts were comparatively low. The counts of micro-organisms were higher on the surface of the sample than in the interior. A number of organisms which would produce surface taint were isolated from defective butter, but were always found in small number. *Achromobacter putrefaciens* which regularly produced the defect in unsalted butter was first isolated from conadian butter (Hammer, 1946). The organism was greatly restrained by the use of moderate amounts of salts or by the use of butter culture.

(e) *Other Defects:* In addition to the defects already described, a number of other defect develop on holding, some of which are slightly different from those already described, while others very considerably. Organisms of Escherichia-Aerobacter group, particularly some Aerobacter species. Some times produce unclean flavours in butter. Hammer and Yale (1932) found that in butter both low temperature and salt concentration have marked influence in inhibiting the growth of the organisms of this group.

Colour changes also occur in butter as a result of growth of many organisms viz. Moulds, yeasts and serratia species producing different colours. These colour changes occur more readily in unsalted than in salted butter because of the growth inhibitory action of salt. Mould growth on butter generally results in an unsightly appearance and off-flavours, developing mould spots frequently during summer months.

In serious spoilages, the sports may penetrate into the butter to a considerable depth. According to Thom and shaw (1915) mould growth to butter is of three general types:

1. Orange-Yellow (red) area, with a submerged growth of riycleium, attributed or *Oidium lacits*.
2. Smudged or dirty green areas, either entirely sub-merged or with some surface growth. These are produced by alternaria and cladosparium.
3. Green surface colonies, which are produced by penicillium or more rarely Aspergillus upon the butter causing decomposition.

Several genra and species of moulds capable of growing in butter and causing the above defects have also been reported by Hammer (1946).

Bacteriological Analysis

A. Sampling

1. *Sampling of Butter*: Smaples of creamery butter were collected from some of the local dairies in Roorkee. Since butter is usualy sold in packets wrapped in butter paper, they were taken as such in fifty gram size packs and taken to the laboratory. The sample was thoroughly mixed by means of a sterile spatula and transferred to a sterile ground glass stopped bottle.

2. *Sampling of Cream*: Samples of cream used by the different dairies were collected dairies were collected separately in sterlized stoppered glass containers. These were analysed without any delay for accurate results.

3. *Sampling of Wash Water*: The analysis of wash water is important aspect. The types of organisms derived from water probably affects the keeping quality more than those derived from cream. Therefore, an organism from added water is more serious from the stand point of deterioration.

4. *Sampling of Air*: Air contamination in butter manufacture is important since it is exposed to air for a long duration during backing. For this plated petri-plates for growth of bacteria, yeasts and moulds were exposed to environment of dairies for a period of few minutes and incubated for 24-48 hours and their colonies counted.

B. Preliminary Examination of Samples

The physical condition, flavour and other features were noted down in respect of each sample. In order to get an idea about the predominant organisms present in the butter samples, microscopic examination of the smears taken from the sample was carried out immediately. For this a representative portion of the sample was melted carefully by heating it to 45°C and ten ml. transferred means of a warm wet pipette to a sterile test tube. The test tube was closed with a sterile rubber stopper. The test tube inverted andm in this position centrifuged till the serum separated from the fat. The tube was then kept inverted in the refrigerator for the fat to solidify. The serum free fat was then transferred to another sterile test tube shaken well and a smear taken, which was stained with Borax-ethylene blue.

C. Bacteriological Analysis

The sample of butter were examined for total counts, combined yeasts and mould counts and other types according to the procedure outlined below:

1. *Sterlization of Glasswere and Equipment*: All the glass-ware like pipettes, dilution tubes and petridishes used in the experiment were thoroughly cleaned, dried and sterlized in an oven at 160°C for not less than two hours before use.

2. *Preparation of Dilutions*: For preparation of dilutions use sterile quarter strength Ringer's solution was made.

Ringer's Solution (Quarter Strength):

NaCl	0.9 g
KCl	0.042 g
$CaCl_2 . 8H_2O$	0.048 g
$NaCHO_3$	0.02 g
Distilled water	400 ml

Sterlize by auto claving at 121°C for 20 minutes.

3. *Preparation of Samples*: The sample jars containing the samples of butter to be tested were placed in a water bath between

40 and 45°C and rotated until the butter was of thin creamy consistency. The time required for the sample to reach the creamy consistency was not allowed to exceed fifteen minutes.

4. *Preparing and Pouring the Plates*: The dilution flask containing the sample was rotated twenty-five times, the time interval not eceeeding seven seconds. The dilutions were prepared by taking out 1ml. of this mixture and transferring to 9 ml of warm sterile saline. At appropriate dilution, withdraw 1 ml of the dilution touching the tip of the pipette against the side of the dilution flask to remove excess adhering to the outside and the contents were transferred to the petri-dishes. While transferring to the petri-dishes, the end of the pipette was held at an angle of 45° against the petri-dish and the diluted sample was allowed to drain from the graduation mark to the apparent rest point in the tip of the pipette and then touched once against a dry spot on the glass. Care was taken to raise the petri-dish cover only just enough to insert the pipette.

To each of the prepared plate, 10 ml of molten agar was added at 45°C and immediately the medium and inoculum were mixed by shaking in circular movements for 5-10 seconds. Then the plates are allowed to set, inverted and incubated at the appropriate temperature.

5. *Preparation of Media*: The following media were employed for the enumeration of different organisms.

Plate Count Agar: General viable count of bacteria is normally carried out on a non-selective nutrient medium such as platecount agar (also known as tryptone Glucose Yeast Extract Agar).

Tryptone	5.0 g
Yeast Extract	2.5 g
Dextrose	1.0 g
Agar	15.0 g
Distilled water	1 litre
pH	7.0

The use of nutrient agar is avoided since, it does not allow the growth of certain types of bacteria particularly streptococcin which may be found quite frequently in food.

For standard plate count incubate plates for 48 hours at 37°C. Coliform Bacteria were counted on violet red bile agar.

olet Red Bile Agar

Yeast Extract	3.0 g
Peptone	7.0 g
Bile Salt (Sodium taurocholate)	1.5 g
NaCl	5.0 g
Lactose	10.0 g
Agar	15.0 g
Neutral red	0.3 g
Crystal violet	0.002 g
Distilled water	1 litre
pH	7.4

MacConeky's broth and MacConey's Agar are not satisfactory media for the detection and enumeration of coliform organisms in milk. One of the most reliable methods uses violet red bile agar in pour plate counts.

After agar had solidified, 2 to 4 ml. of the same medium is again poured over it in order to eliminate the possibility of the solid mixture in order to eliminate the possibility of the occurrence of a typical surface colonies of coliforms, (American Standard Methods, 1941).

Incubate at 37°C for 24 hours. After incubation count the number of dark red colonies. Normally typical coliform colonies will be 0.5 mm or more in diameter and show evidence of the precipitation of bile salts in the medium immediately surrounding the colonies.

China Blue Agar, was used for counting acid producers. The medium was prepared according to the following composition (Jorgensen *et al.*, 1939):

Lemco	1 g
Bacto-Peptone	5 g
Dextrose	1 g
Frsh skimmed milk	20 ml
Shred agar	15 g
China Blue (Grubler salt)	2.5 ml

(Saturated aqueous solution)

Distilled water	1 litre
pH	7.0

Acid producers are identified by the formation of very fine blue coloured colonies.

Yeasts and moulds were counted on potato dextrose agar:

Potato	200 g
Dextrose	20 g
Agar agar	15 g
Distilled water	1 litre
pH	4.5

The pH of the medium was adjusted to 3.5 ± 0.1 by adding. 17 ml of a sterile 0.1% aqueous solution of tartaric acid for every ten ml, of medium immediately before pouring on plates. (American Standard Methods, 1941)

6. *Plate Counts*: After the plates were poured, they were incubated for 5 days at 30°C except in the case of coliforms which were counted at the end of twenty four hours incubation, since further incubation of the plates gave rise to the growth of certain non coliforms like micrococcii and pinpoint colonies of thermoduric streptococci, giving inaccurate plate counts. All results of plate counts were calculated form the average of the duplicates of each dilution counted. Occasionaly the china Blue Agar became completely bleached after incubationdue to the growth of organisms, thus making it difficult to take differential counts. In such cases only total count was recorded.

Observation and Results

A study was made find out the keeping quality and changes in the microflora of butter at refrigeration temperature (9±2°C) among the dairies located at Roorkee. Results obtained from this survey study are descrbed here below.

The samples of cram and wash water were collected from various dairies of Roorkee and analysed without any delay. The air samples were taken in duplicates and total counts calculated by taking the mean of the plates. The cream was found to be separated from the milk with the aid of cream separator without being pasteurised. This came out to be the main reason for high plate counts obtained.

On microscopic examination, the samples (A, B, C, D and E) showed a predominance of streptococci, lactobacilli and rod forms occasionally. Yeasts and moulds were seldom seen although they grew subsequently in the plate cultures.

The numbers of different group bacteria, coliforms, yeasts and moulds counted in respect of cream wash water and air samples are indicated in Tables 5.1, 5.2 and 5.3.

The Coliform content in cream came out to be exceptionally high in some dairien. Yeasts and mould acounts and bacterial counts and bacterial counts for air samples taken in dairy environment showed a significant number.

A study was also conducted on changes in microflora of salted and unsalted creamery butters of Roorkee dairies. The samples were subjects to storage at refrigeration temperature and examined initially and at intervals of 3, 7, 10, 15 and 30 days for general appearance, acidity, total bacterial counts as well as counts of coliforms and cambined yeast and moulds counts.

The colour and texture of the experimental creamery butters were satisfactory at the commencement of storage. The samples had a flat taste. As the period of storage advanced, mould growth became visible at the surface of all the samples with the formation of various colour spots. In some places the moulds seemed to have penetrated inside the butter. Although the flavour became unpleasant and slightly mouldy, it could not exactly be indentified with any characteristic odours.

The results of studies of the storage of different samples of experimental salted and unsalted butters are given in Tables 5.4, 5.5, 5.6 and 5.7.

Abbrevations Used

A: National dairy
B: Shiv dairy
C: Malik dairy
D: Maheshwari dairy
E: Milan dairy

Table 5.1

Total and differential counts of microflora of cream samples used in the preparation of creamery butters

(Counts per ml)

Sample Number	Standard Plate Count	Coliform Count
A	54,000	1,17,000
B	1,39,000	1,60,000
C	92,000	1,79,000
D	40,000	73,000
E	87,000	1,10,000

Table 5.2

Total and differential counts of microflora of wash water used in preparation of creamery butter

(Counts per ml)

Sample Number	Standard Plate Count	Coliform Count
A	89,000	23,000
B	27,000	98,000
C	1,18,000	71,000
D	63,000	66,000
E	47,000	32,000

Table 5.3

Total and differential counts of microflora of air samples taken in diary plants

(Counts per ml)

Sample Number	Total bacterial Count	Total Yeast and Mould Count
A	271	318
B	408	273
C	317	581
D	123	215
E	392	374

Table 5.4
Changes in microbial content of unsalted creamery butter sample "A" of Roorkee dairy during storage at refregeration temperature
(Counts per ml)

Time of Storage (Days)	Total Plate Counts	Coliform Counts	Acid Producers Counts	Combined Yeast and mould Counts
0	33,000	7,200	63,000	57,000
3	2,03,000	47,000	93,000	82,000
7	3,45,000	1,12,000	99,000	3,40,000
10	6,90,000	87,000	1,25,000	7,63,000
15	7,02,000	35,000	1,32,000	7,98,000
30	1,22,000	600	1,68,000	5,84,000

Table 5.5
Changes in microbial content of unsalted creamery butter sample "B" on storage at refregeration temperature
(Counts per ml)

Time of Storage (Days)	Total Plate Counts	Coliform Counts	Acid Producers Counts	Combined Yeast and mould Counts
0	64,000	700		5000
3	97,000	5,600	52,000	38,500
7	1,45,000	15,400	1,17,000	1,75,000
10	5,90,000	12,050	1,45,000	2,22,000
15	7,25,000	3,500	1,70,000	1,64,000
30	6,78,000	800	2,01,000	79,000

Similarly, Ghodekar (1969), Hemavathy et al. (1974), Sharma and Zariwala (1978), Sachdeva and Rajorhia (1982), Vijaybhader at al. (1983), Garg *et al.* (1984), Patel (1986), and Rajorhia and Sen (1987) all have reported a lower average as well as lower range of values of protein in burfi and/or peda.

Thus on the basis of protein lodge, burfi and peda are placed in descending order.

Table 5.6
**Changes in microbial content of unsalted creamery butter sample
"C" stored at refregeration temperature**

(Counts per ml)

Time of Storage (Days)	Total Plate Counts	Coliform Counts	Acid Producers Counts	Combined Yeast and mould Counts
0	73,000	5,000	14,000	—
3	1,52,000	55,000	17,000	12,400
7	1,76,000	1,29,000	1,05,000	38,500
10	3,20,000	1,06,000	1,37,000	1,75,000
15	2,27,000	63,000	1,50,000	1,72,000
30	1,95,000	3,000	1,57,000	1,15,000

Table 5.7
**Changes in microbial content of salted creamery butter sample "D"
during storage at refregeration temperature**

(Counts per ml)

Time of Storage (Days)	Total Plate Counts	Coliform Counts	Acid Producers Counts	Combined Yeast and mould Counts
0	52,000	850	11,500	2,500
3	90,000	3000	15,050	12,300
7	1,06,000	12,400	35,000	50,000
10	1,25,000	38,000	91,000	1,07,000
15	2,58,000	24,030	1,06,000	1,25,000
30	1,73,000	2,500	1,42,000	87,000

Discussion

Micro-organisms play a significant role in the development of
off-flavour and other defects and in bringing about the
decomposition of butter in various ways, considerable importance
is attached to the numbers of microflora (bacteria, yeasts and
moulds) present in the material. Due to the selective environment
offered by butter for bacterial growth, as indicated above, more
emphasis may be laid on the types than on the numbers of

organisms occuring in it. There has therefore, been considerable controversy regarding the significance to be attached with the numerical distribution of microflora in butter and accordingly there have been no bacterial standards prescribed for grading and quality of market butter as the case of milk. A number of workers have however tried to asses the variation in the total bacterial counts and numbers of specific groups of organisms like coliforms, lipolytic micro-organisms, yeasts and mould etc., as a possible means of estimating the sanitary conditions during butter manufacture and it's probable keeping quality of storage.

The samples of cream, wash waters and air (Tables 5.1, 5.2 and 5.3) to asses keeping quality of butters of local Roorkee daries indicates the prevailing unhygenic conditions. In the case of cream samples being analysed, coliform content is very higher varying from 70,000 to 1,80,000 and from 22,000 to nearly 100,000 in case of wash water. A number of strains of coliform bacteria (Pont, 1935) are isolated causing rapid and serious deterioration. The total bacterial count is less than 1,40,000 per ml. The sources of contamination of cream (Elliker, 1941) includes dust, dirt, manure and unclean utensils.

Similarly preponderance of yeast and moulds in air samples and cream samples analysed may contaminate the butters during the course of their preparation, handling and their exposure for sale. In general, low grade samples of butter (Redfield, 1922) show high yeast counts. Olson and Hammer, (1934) studied the numbers of bacterial, yeasts and moulds falling from the air and found that amongst the three, bacteria were the most numerous and yeast the least. Some of the samples examined in the present study showed appreciable moulds like Penicillium, cladosporium and other types.

Many unhygenic practices were observed by the author on visiting the various dairies areas. The cream meant for preparing butter in some cases are obtained with the aid of cream separators without pasteurising it at all. This is supposed to be the main reason behind high counts obtained. Secondly the lumps of butter are separated with the bare hands by workers of dairy plants. Moreover no restriction was implemented to restrict air currents in dairy plants in sue course of butter preparation.

Sometime as numerical distribution of microflora in butter is concerned, the anamolies involved in judging the sanitary conditions of manufacture or keeping quality of butter is by means of total number of bacteria present in them. Since coliform organisms, yeasts are moulds are generally external contaminants, their presence in large number may be taken to indicate unhygenic methods of manufacture and handling. The importance of sanitary methods in the production of butters cannot be therefore under emphasised.

In the experimental creamery butter samples (Table 5.4, 5.5, 5.6 and 5.7), the acidity rises slowly. There is however a greater increase of acidity in the unsalted series than in the salted ones at the end of thirty days storage (Rahn, Brown and Smitth, 1909). The acidity of the unsalted series is more than that shown by the corresponding salted series. This may be due to the inhibitory effect of salt on the activities of organisms responsible for increasing the acidity (Macy, 1927 and Guthrie, Scheib and Stark, 1936).

The coliform counts go on increasing upto 15 days and then fall off in the case of salted butter while in case of unsalted butter, the organisms fall off ofter seven days (Loftus, Hills, Scharp and Bellair, 1934). This difference is probably due to the higher acidities developed in the unsalted series during different stages of production. There is no difinite relationship between increase in acidity and total bacterial count.

In both salted and unsalted butters, the total counts show a considerable increase from the beginning upto 15 days after which they then fall off. Yeast and mould counts rise slowly upto 15 days and off, but in case of unsalted samples the increase is greatest and corresponds to increased development of acidity. Simultaneously the colour defects and off-flavours formed in the sample which have been reffered to previously became more pronounced. In the case of unsalted butter, therefore, an increase in total counts as well as the combined yeast and mould counts appear to bear some relationship with rise in acidity. Addition of salt is inhibitory to microbial activity and to some excent, resulting in the improvement of keeping quality.

Considering the small numbers of organisms encountered in the samples, it may however be presumed that the types of organisms are more important than their numbers in the deterioration of butter. This may be observed clearly in salted and unsalted samples where there is development of high acidity with a corresponding increase in the numbers of bacteria or combined yeast and mould counts.

Therefore, it would appear that there was no definite correlation between total counts and development of acidity during storage, although the effect of bacterial activity on the deterioration of butter is seen particularly in unsalted butter samples. High acidity as well as salting had a retarding influence on the bacterial growth. Combined yeast and mould counts showed correlation with the rise in acidity. The results also show the effect of high initial acidity on the rate of it's development during the storage of butter.

Summary

1. From a consideration of the factors affecting the quality of salted and unsalted creamery butters, the importance of microbial activity in the spiloage of butter is discussed. The relative importance of numbers and of types of microflora occuring in butters has been indicated.

2. A study of microflora of samples of salted creamery butter and unsalted creamery butter has been reported.
   As a result of the numbers and of the different groups of micro-organisms in butters it was observed that:

   (i) The total bacterial count of unsalted creamery butters was higher in comparision to that of salted creamery butters.

   (ii) The coliform count of salted butters was less than unsalted creamery butters.

   (iii) The unsalted creamery butters registered higher count of lipolytic organisms than the salted creamery butters.

   (iv) The increase in acidity was found to be in relation with an increase in number of yeasts and moulds in salted and unsalted creamery butter.

   (v) Amongst the different groups of bacteria counted in all the types butters, the acid producers were the largest in numbers.

3. The reasons of the differences between salted and unsalted creamery butters are discussed. It has been suggested that:

(i)   The creamery butter is likely to be contaminated during manufacture and handling unless very strict sanitary precautions are followed;

(ii) The numbers of coliforms are lower in salted creamery butters to that of unsalted creamery butters due to the inhibitory effect of sodium chloride on species of coliforms.

4. The significance of these observations on the control of the quality of butter has been indicated.

5. A detailed examination of the morphological, cultural and biochemical characteristics of the organisms isolated from the creamery butters has been carried out. It was found that:

   The *Lactobacilli* were the most predominant types in butter samples, other types being *Streptococcus*, *Micrococci*, *Coliforms* and *Aerobic spore formers*. Some samples of creamery butters also showed the presence of organisms belonging to *Pseudomonas*, *Serratia* and *Achromobacter* genra and responsible for production of taints.

6. The keeping quality of Roorkee dairy butters has been discussed:

   (i)   Since coliform organisms, yeasts and moulds are generally external contaminants their presence in large numbers may be taken to indicate unhygenic methods of manufacture and handling.

   (ii) During the course of this study, it was observed that use of unpasteurised cream and separation of butter, (after being churned) bare handed by workers, is the main malpractice carried out in the local dairies.

7. The changes in the microflora of area dairy butter during storage has been discussed. It was found that when butter was stored at refrigeration temperature:

   (i)   There was no preciese correlation between the development of acidity during storage and the total bacterial count of the butter.

(ii) A high initial acidity of butter restrained bacterial growth to some extent, and

(iii) The increase in the development of acidity of butters was related to the increase of the combined yeast and mould counts of the butters.

8. The significance of these findings in the spoilage of butter during storage are discussed.

9. The organisms isolated from different samples of butters were characterized and identified as :

Lactobacilus Species: *L. acidophilus, L. plantarum, L. bulgaricus* and *L. casei.*

Streptococcus Species: *S. durans, S. lactis, S. cremoris* and *S. diacetyl-aromaticus.*

Micrococcus Species: *M. citreus, M. flavus,* and *M. albus.*

Aerobic Spore Formers: *B. subtilis, B. pumilis,* (Bacillus species)

Coliforms: *E. Coli, Aerobacter aerogens*

Intermediate and Irregular types.

Taint Producers: Belonging generally to *Pseudomonas, serratia* and *Achromobacter* genera.

Yeasts: Mostly asporogenous yeasts, few pink yeasts probably belonging to *Rhodotorulaceae.*

Moulds: Species of *Penicillium, Cladosporium Alternaria, Mucor, Rhizopus* and *Fusarium.*

6

FERMENTED MILK

Milk fermentations for processing of milk into cultured milk products for increasing the shelf life and having different flavour and texture characteristics have been practiced in different parts of the world. Milk has been processed into cheese, kefir, *dahi*, koumiss and various other fermented milks. Yoghurt is one such fermented, slightly acid, semi-solid or stirred cultured milk food that derives its modern vogue from the balkons where it has long been popular, Youghurt is a product made from milk that has been heat treated, with its solid content increased that is then fermented by means of specific organism, namely, a complementary combination of *Str. thermophilus* and *L. bulgaricu* to bring about flavour and aroma development, physical change and an acidity of at least 0.7 g of lactic acid/100g of yoghurt.

In the business of fermented milk products lactic starters occupy key position as the success or failure of such products is directly related to the type of starter used. The first scientific study on lactic starters was carried out by Danish Bacteriologist Storch in 1890.

1. YOGHURT STARTERS

Traditionally production of yoghurt must involve a fermentation of milk by a mixed culture of *Str. Thermophilus* and *L. bulgaricus*. The validity of this idea is supported by Kon (1959), although Davis (1973) suggested that *L. bulgaricus* and any other suitable lactic acid bacterium still give rise to yoghurt. This latter approach has, of course, some justification, because if is generally agreed that the desiraable flavour and aroma of yoghurt is derived from the presence of *L. bulgaricus*. However, two points can be put forward in favour of Kon's view. First that *Str. Thermophilus* is almost universally employed in commercial practice and second that there is evidence of an interaction between *Str. Thermophilus* and *L. bulgaricus* leading to the improved development of the latter (Galesloot *et al.* (1968): Verenga *et al.*, (1968); Robinson and Tamime, (1975).

Several workers [Pette and Lolkema, (1950); Davis, (1956); (1967); Crawford, 1962; Humphrey and Plunken, (1969) and Davis, (1971)] have reported that the conventional yoghurt of dairy consumption contains approximately equal number of *Str. thermophilus* and *L. bulgaricus*. A mixed culture of *Str. thermophilus* and *L. bulgaricus* has been satisfactorily used in the yoghurt making from concentrated milk (Buandgaard *et al.*, (1972); Donnelly *et al.*, (1977); Davis *et al.* (1977).

Str. thermophilus which is considered to be a essential bacterial component of a yoghurt culture, has a high sensitivity to bacterial inhibitors and often causes difficulties in the yoghurt manufacture (Teply, 1970). A new mixed culture composed of pexiococcus *acidilactici*, *Str. Thermophilus* and *L. bulgaricus* has been successfully employed in yoghurt pkeparation from milic containing inhibitors in Czechoslovak dairy factories since 1969. Davis *et al.*, (1971) describe methods for enumerating the viable *streptococci* and *lactobacilli* in mixed cultures, used for the production of yoghurt.

Johannson (1975) explanied the starter production process and reported the principle characteristics and various appalications of different species of bacteria most commonly used as starters for the manufacture of fermented milk products like yoghurt. The validity of specifying *Str. thermophilus* and *L. bulgaricus* in the mixed cultures of yoghurt had been explained by Robinson and Tamime (1975, 1976).

In the past six or seven years, there had been several comprehensive review articles on the modern developments in the behaviour characteristics and technology of *Str. thermophilus* and *L. bulgaricus* in the production of yoghurt (Mocquot and Hurre, (1970); Tamer (1973); and Tamime and Robinson, (1976).

2. ASSOCIATIVE GROWTH OF *STR. THERMOPHILUS* AND *L. BULGARICUS*

The two organisms, *Str. Thermophilus* and *L. bulgaricus* have a complementary relationship in the preparation of yoghurt. The streptococci grow first, prepare the way for the lactobacilli by removing the oxygen which otherwise can lead to the production of toxic hydrogen peroxide.

The growth of streptococci in yoghurt making is slowed down with liberation of amino acids and lowering of pH by lactobacilli. Acidity development was mainly due to *L. bulgaricus*, the streptococci being inhibited at the lower pH. At 0.9% acidity, the ratio was 1:1 (Hymphreys and Plumkett, 1969).

Kurmann (1966) observed that incubation of yoghurt starters at 42°C after inculation at a rate of 2% maintained the starter ratioa of cocci : rods at 1:1 and the acidifying capacity of mixed culture could be maintained best at refrigerated temperature (Tamime and Robinson, (1976).

The studies conducted by Pette and Lolkema (1950 a, b) have shown that the more rapid acid production by mixed culture of *Str. thermophilus* and *L. bulgaricus* was attributable to water soluble, heat stable growth factors for the streptococci, produced by lactobacilli. They also indicated that these factors were amino acids and the valine was the most stimulatory one. But Bautista *et al.* (1966) have found that histidine and glycine were mainly responsible for the improved growth of *Str. thermophilus*.

Miller and Kandler (1964) reported that free amino acid contents of yoghrut samples from *Str. thermophilus* and *L. bulgaricus* contained more free serine and threonine than other amino acids. In a subsequent paper (1964a); they determined free amino acids quantitatively in the diffusable material obtained from milk and yoghurt. The high proteolytic nature of *L. bulgaricus* caused considerable increase in free amino acids, which were subsequently utilized for the growth of *Str. thermophilus*.

According to Galesloot *et al.* (1968), it is *Str. thermophilus* which stimulated *L. bulgaricus* by producing a growth factor in milk which was equal to or can be replaced by formic acid. This stimulation could only be demonstrated in moderately heated milk and not in the sterilized milk, which contained formic acid elaborated by the heating process. They further indicated that Pette and Lolkema (1950a, b) and Bautista *et al.* (1966) had failed to observe the stimulation by *Str. thermophilus* , because they had used severely heated milk.

Veringa *et al.* (1968) conducted a number of experiments in order to isolate and identify stimulatory substanc, which was found to be volatile with steam and extractable with ether. Volatile fatty acids produced by *Str. thermophilus* were isolated and separated by means of chromtographic techniques. The stimulation tests on the separated acid, furnished sufficient evidence that the substance which stimulated *L. bulgaricus* and was elaborated by *Str. thermophilus* in yoghurt milk was formic acid.

Growth of *Str. thermophilus* in mixed culture was enhanced during the exponential phase (Moon and Reinbold, 1976) than when grown alone. *L. bulgaricus* liberated Seitz-filterable compounds during its growth that stimulated the growth of *Str. thermophilus*. These compounds were believed to be responsible for commensal response observed in the mixed cultures.

Shanker and Davis (1978) confirmed the obseivations of Vergina *et al.* (1968) that formate was an important stimulant for *L. bulgaricus* produced by *Str. thermophilus*. Since milk for yoghurt making contained little formate, production of this compound by *Str. thermophilus* was essential. They further observed that production of formate and acetaldehyde by *Str. thermophilus* was found to be strain variable, emphasizing the imporance of culture selection.

Higashio *et al.* (1978) studied that growth factros of *L. bulgaricus* produced by *Str. thermophilus* were formic and pyruvic acid and these two acids showed a syanergistic effect on the stimulation of acid production and grwoth of *L. bulgaricus*.

3. BIOCHEMICAL ACTIVITY OF YOGHURT BTARTRRB :

(a) Acid Production

One of the most important points in mixed cultures of *Str. thermophilus* and *L. bulgaricus* in to deliver the yoghurt al the best acidity. A very careful control of the acid production is necessary because the yoghurt organisms grow rapidly and the titratable acidity at the point of clotting will vary with different types of milk (Wilkowske, 1954 and Davis, 1956).

The role of lactic acid starters in the production of acid in fermented milks like yoghurt, has been earlier studied by several workers Laxminarayana *et al*, (1952); Mabbit, 1961 and Marth, 1962).

Gllilland and Olson (1963) studied the rates of acid production by milka cultures in various fractions of milk. The cultures produced acid more rapidly in the whole milk than in skim milk. Further the culture lactic starters propagated in a mixture of skim milk and butter milk produced acid rapidly than in either produced alone.

Ashton (1963) suggesed the incubation of *Str. thermophilus* to a low acidity point and of *L. bulgaricus* to high acidity point in the manufacture of youghurt. Bautista *et al.* (1966) and reported that the beneficial effect was essentially limited to the gradual accumulation of factors in *L. bulgaricus* culture that promoted more rapid acid production by *Str. thermophilus.*

Iyengar *et al.* (1967) noticed considerable differences in the rate of acid production by *Str. thermophilus* and *L. bulgaricus* in different types of milk. *Str. thermophilus* produced more acid in soy milk (Hary and Jackson, 1967) and it has been confirmed by other workers (Kim and Shin, 1971). *L. bulgaricus* and *Str. thermophilus* mixed with *L. bulgaricus* had been frequently used to prepare fermented products from soy milk (Wang *et al.*, 1974).

Thomas *et al.* (1966) observed acid production by various lactic cultures in cow and buffalo milk. A marked increase in acid production was noticed in the buffalo as compared to cow milk.

Lee and Price (1969) studied the lactic acid prodution by *L. bulgaricus* in milk and tomato juice both.

Dutta *et al.* (1971) recorded high amounts of acid production by *L. bulgaricus* which was quite significant in view of the important role of this organism together with *Str. thermophilus.* In the preparation of yoghurt. In a subsequent paper (1971) they reported the effect of day-to-day variations in reconstituted milk prepared from different brands of milk powder and in skim milk obtained from milk of different species on the activity of *Str. thermophilus* and *L. bulgaricus.* Preliminary studies with the selected strains of *Str. thermophilus* and *L. bulgaricus* revealed that high acid production occurred in mixed culture due to enhanced growth of streptococci (Moon and Renbold, 1976).

Accolas *et al.* (1977) reported the acid producing properties of different strains of *Str. thermophilus* and *L. bulgaricus* in pure and mixed-strain cultures. Mixed cultures always produced more acid than the corresponding pure culture.

Singh and Ranganathan (1978) observed acid production by L. *bulgaricus* in different types of milk. They found more acid production by the lactobacillie in buffalo than in cow milk.

(b) Flavour Production

In fermented food products like yoghurt, aroma and flavour are the main determinants of palatability and therefore, of sales. Several review articles have been published on different aspects of flavour production by starter bacteria in recent years (Galesloot, 1962; Keenan and Bills, 1968; Robinson and Tamime, 1975). In the present review, considerations are given to some of the important flavour compounds produced by yoghurt starters.

Yoghurt is invariably prepared by using a mixed culture of *Str. thermophilus* and L. *bulgaricus* and the reason for using this combination was that it had been found to give the best results from the flavour point of view and Lolkema, (1950), Davis, (1956).

Acetaldehyde, which is the principle flavour component of yoghurt Pette and Lolkema, (1950) is reported to be produced from number of compounds, among them being lactose Seneca *et al.*, 1950), valine acetylphosphate and pyruvate (Lee and Jago, 1966). Schulz and Things (1954) reported colorimetric determination of acetaldehyde in yoghurt starter organisms, which was suitable for assessing the flavour development.

Davis (1956) reported that *Str. thermophilus* produced diacetyl during its growth in mixed culture of yoghurt. Dutta *et al.* (1971) reported that no diacetyl was produced by L. *bulgaricus* in steam-sterilized milk.

Galesloot (1960) reported that diacetyl was formed through oxidation of acetoin and under aerobic conditions acetoin and diacetyl were produced from acetolactic acid, while under anaerobic conditions, only aceton was formed. Rasic and Milanovic (1966) found that pure strain yoghurt cultures produced a little amount of diacetyl in milk.

Dutta *et al.* (1972) recorded increase volatile acid production by *Str. thermophilus* and L. *bulgaricus* with an increase in citric acid concentration. A relationship was established between the production of hydrogen Sulphide and volatile Fatty acids Terkazaryan, (1973).

Yu *et al.* (1974) studied that different strains of *Str. thermophilus* and *L. bulgaricus* exhibited variations. In the production of soluble fatty acids in different types of milk. Yu and Nakanishi (1975) noticed that there was a pronounced effect of milk fat on the production of valatile carbonyl compouds by mixed lactic starters.

Harvery (1960) reported on acetaldehyde production by lactic streptococci in cultured milk products. Lindasy *et al.* (1965) studied that excessive acetaldehyde production was correlated with "green flavour" of yoghurt cultures. Lindsay and Day (1965) observed that concentration of acetaldehyde and diacetyl in lactic cultures determined the intensity of flavour. The quantitative production of dactyl and acetaldehyde in lactic cultures has been extensively studied Pack *et al.*, (1964); Lindsay and Day, (1965); Lindsay *et al.*, (1965).

Bottazzi and Delluglio (1967) determined the diacetyl and acetaldehyde ratio in milk cultures of *Str. thermophilus*. They compared different cultures in skim milk with regard to acetaldehyde and diacetyl production.

Lindsay *et al.* (1965) evaluated various strains of lactic cultures for the substances which contributed flavour to the fermented milk preparations. Diacetyl, acetaldehyde and acetoin were estimated primarily.

Speckman and Collins (1968) showed that two distinct pathway were involved in the production of acetaldehyde directly, acetoin or diacetyl.

Bottazzi and Vescova (1969) correlated the activity of lactic cultures with the production of carbonyl compunds during the manufacture of yoghurt. Yashima *et al.* (1970) and Henry (1972) reported the acetone production by hetero-fermentative lactobacilli, but this had not been examined for lactic streptococci.

Bills *et al.* (1972) observed the influence of sucrose on the production of acetaldehyde by *Str. thermophilus* and *L. bulgaricus*. Jonsson and Petterson (1977) compared the activity of different lactic cultures for the citric acid fermentation with regard to – acetolactate. Lees and Jago (1977) and Robinson (1977) studied the biochemical performance of lactic acid bacteria in the formation of acetaldehyde, which was an indicator of flavour intensity in yoghurt.

Recently, Abrahmsen *et al.* (1978) observed no significant differences in volatile aromatic compounds by yoghurt bacteria an goat and cow milk.

(c) Proteolytic Activity

The proteolytic activity of lactic acid bacteria in milk was reported by Von Freudenreich as early as in 1896. Various lactic cultures were grown in different types of milk in order to elucidate their proteolytic patterns using different methods.

Sterile chalk milk cultures of these organisms were known to bring about a substantial increase in soluble nitrogen content.

After examining the proteolytic activity of nearly 200 strains of thermophilic lactobacilli isolated from milk samples, Braz and Allen (1938) found that only a few strains exhibited very high proteolytic activity. The above workers concluded that there was no correlation between proteolytic activity and acid production by the cultures. Recently, Akopyan and Swakhanyan (1972) had als arrived at the same conclusion while studying the proteolytic activity and acid forming ability of several strains of streptococci.

Sasaki and Nakae (1958) isolated 30 strains of lactic acid bacteria from raw milk and reported that five were strongly proteolytic. In a subsequent paper, Sasaki and Nakee (1959) further reported the proteolytic activity of 258 strains of lactic acid bacteria by estimating the amount of tryosine liberated during incubation.

Proteolytic activity of lactic streptococci at refrigerated storage conditions was studied by Cowman and Speck (1962). Pronounced reduction was noted in regard to the proteolytic activity of growing toluene-treated cells after the first one or two days of storage at 2-4°C. In a later paper, Cowman and Speck (1963) reported drastic reduction in proteolytic activity at –20°C, while storage at temperature of –296°C reduced enzymatic activity only slaightly.

It has been noted that lactobacilli possessed greater proteolytic abilities as compared to streptococci Zalaskhko and Molachova, (1967); Searles *et al.*, (1970). Maksimova (1968) studied the proteolytic activity of various streptococci with the object of using some of these strains in the preparation of cultured milk products. Some species of lactobacilli such as *bulgaricus* were found more proteolytic than streptococci.

Nachev (1969) studied the pattern of amino acid production by 125 strains of L. *bulgaricus* which had been isolated from commercial and home made yoghurts in Bulgaria. The cultures were grouped into three categories on the basis of amino acid analysis. The first category comprised of 118 strains and these were characterized by liberation of leucine, gluamtic acid, asparagine, proline and absence of aminobutyric acid, alanine, and tryptophan. The second category which included 6 strains was distinguished by the absence of glutamiac acid, while the third group which had only strain was characterized by the presence of tryptophan.

A few strains of L. *bulgaricus* showing moderate proteolytic activity were isloated from commercial and domestic yoghurt sample Nachev, (1969).

Formisano *et al.* (1970) studied the proteolytic acitivity of yoghurt starters with a view to use this information in the manufacture of yoghurt. Centrifugal supernatants recovered from lysozyme-treated cells of L. *bulgaricus* and **Str. thermophilus** were used for proteolytic activity, which was found to decrease with the reduction in pH from 7.0 to 4.0. Maximum proteolytic activity was observed in L. *bulgaricus* and compared to *Str. thermophilus* or a combination for *Str. thermophilus* with L. *bulgaricus*.

Crudzinskaya and Koroleva (1970) have reported various changes in the amino acid spectrum in milk cultures of *Str. thermophilus* and L. *bulgaricus*. The streptococci liberated glumtamic acid, glycine, threonine, alanine, tyrosine, while lactobacilli released glutamic acid, histidine, arginine, tryosine, phenylalanine, leucine, cysteine, methionine and valine.

Ter-Kazar'yan (1974) reported that proteolytic activity of lactobcilli was double than that of streptococci, statistically, no significant relationship was found between strain or species and proteolytic activity, when selected strains were evaluated for use in the cheese industry.

Luca (1974) studied the proteolytic changes and amino acid liberation by lactic acid bacteria used in yoghurt manufacture. They found that proteolytic activity of **Str. Thermophilus** was very low and final values for contents of free amino acids were lower than the initial values. On the contrary, L. *bulgaricus* caused considerable liberation of amino acids during its growth.

4. PREPARATION OF YOGHURT

Bulgarian workers have proposed a method for the production of forzen active starters for yoghurt manufacture. The optimum results were obtained by freezing yoghurt starters in liquid nitrogen at 38°C-42°C acidity, when the mixed culture (*Str. thermophilus* and *L. bulgaricus*) were employed in the logarithic growth phase.

Progress report on a method of yoghurt production including slow acidification at 30°C have come from Germany. Use is made of "Yoghurt type 30°C", a slow-acting culture which acidified milk at 30°C, produced an excellent yoghurt of typical flavour and consistency in 19-20 hours. When used in combination with *Str. filant* and an "bioactivator". Visker D, a product of similar flavour but much higher viscosity is produced. When *Leuconostoc citrovorum* is added to produce diacetyl, a yoghurt of superior flavour was obtained.

Naeiriuckz (1972) stressed on the "thermisation" of yoghurt. This treatment was conducted at the later state of manufacture on the finished product before packaging, at a temperature generally below 70°C, depending upon the acidity of the product.

In another report Hinterwaldner, (1971), it is claimed that yoghurt-like products which do not sour during bifidus bacteria in addition to normal starter cultures. Growth promoting agents, like yeast extract or autolysates, very production during incubation.

Martens (1972) studied the effect of some variables on the consistency and flavour of stired yoghurt. The variables studied included variations in fat, order of homogenization, starter used (seven different types), percentage starter inocula, degree ·of stirring rate, cooling temperature, temperature of storage and conditions during transport and distribution.

A dessert product, produced by introducing fruit pulp or puree containing aliguate in solution, into steam of viscous, prefermented milk.

5. SHELIF LIFE OF CULTURED MILKS

Kiermier (1972) reported that cultures milk can be stored for a longer period by second pasteurization of the cultured product at 80°C for 15-20 minutes followed by UHT treatment and subsequent cooling to reduce colour and flavour.

Roiner and Grosserhode (1972) pretended method for producing cultured dairy products having a shelf life upto one year by interrupting the incubation in the incubation in the pH ranges above the isoelectric value by cooling and then adjustment of pH range above isoelectric heating to about 110-120°C for sterilizan.

Manufacture of cultured milk products. Maximum exclusion of microbial contamination, aseptic method of production and pasteurisation of finished products were covered by Kohl (1976).

Rakshy (1966) established that sour products could be pasteurised at rather lower temperatures and for shorter periods as compared to sweet milk products. Experiments confirmed that by heating the cultured products for 30 minutes at 50-55°C increased the keeping quality for at least 3 weeks at 15°C. The destructive effect under such conditions was over 95-99% of the initial flora of such products.

Egli and Egli (1977) advocated that higher pasteurisation temperature at more than or at 90°C , homogenisation of milk, concentration by 10%, addition of 10-12% of sugar, incubation with yoghurt starter at 42-44°C to pH 4.0-4.3, cooling to less than 25°C addition of stabilizers and keeping the product at less than 12°C for 5-7 hrs. After filling into containers with hermetic sealing the product to be autoclaved and cooled under pressure to 10-15°C, kept at 4-6°C for 2-4 day and than stored at room temperature so that the product can be stored without refrigeration upto 6 months without loosing its characteristic taste.

Spoilage of Cultured Milks

Spoilage of *dahi* samples on storage was due to non-lactic contaminants such as spore formers, micrococci, coliforms yeasts, and moulds. These undesirable organisms rapidly increased in number when the starter was weak and the ratio of non-lactic to lactic organism was high. Containers having a large surface of air in contact with the fermented milk accelerated the process of spoilage.

Cultured dairy products are generally spoiled by yeasts and moulds and also by lactic acid bacteria which may cause sour, bitter and cheesy flavours.

Lang and Land (1973) reported that cultured milks normally contain flora other than starter bacteria and the presence of the former may have pronounced adverse effects on the quality of these products and their storage life, particularly the use of moulds and yeast have to be excluded.

7

HYDROGEN PAROXIDE AND FORMALIN ON THE MICROFLORA OF RAW MILK

A. THE LACTOPEROXIDASE SYSTEM AND HYDROGEN PEROXIDE (H_2O_2)

Recent year we know number of non-specific, anti-microbial component that gained increasing interest in the milk contains the lactoperoxidase/thiocyanate/ H_2O_2 system (LPS), which has a broad antibacterial spectrum is one of them. The antibacterial effect of LPS is dependent on the level of its 3 components in milk. The concentration of natural thiocyanate (SCN) and H_2O_2 are considered to be the limiting factors for the antibacterial activity of LPS in milk. Therefore addition of small quantities of SCN and H_2O_2 greatly increase the antibacterial activity of LPS system in milk. In practice this has been used to improve the keeping quality of raw milk particularly where proper cooling is not feasible. This system has been successfully used in reducing spoilage of milk under hot climate.

In 1957 FAO discussed use of H_2O_2 as preservation in his meeting which acknowledged its advantages in the transport of milk when refrigeration facilities are not available in tropical countries. It was concluded that H_2O_2 is one of the best chemical treatments that could be safely use to prevent the spoilage of milk for human consumption. The bactericidal effectiveness of H_2O_2 varies with concentration used, the temperature and duration of treatment, the numbers and types of organisms in

---

*Vide Mahmoud, S.Z. *et al.*, 1984.

milk and their resistance. This was studied by Curren (1940*)
Nambudriped and Iya (1949) and (1951),* Morries (1951),*
Demetre (1959) and Luck (1956) and (1962). The main purpose
of this study ws to evaluate the efficiency of various concentrations
of H_2O_2 as preservatives for milk in comparison to various
concentrations of formaline which is used by many local milk
vendors for milk preservation.

Lactoparoxidase is synthesised within the mammary gland
and is present in high concentration in bivine milk. It oxidized
thiocyanate (SCN) in presence of H_2O_2 to an unstable oxidation
product, hypothiocyante (OSCN) which is bactericidal for entirc
pathogens. The system damages the inner membrane causins
leakage and cessation of uptake of nutrient, leading eventually
to death of the organisms and lysis.

Addition of H_2O_2 to milk improved its keeping quality by
destroying or inactivating bacterial population. While untreated
milk samples did not usually keep sweet for greater than 6
Hours at room temperature addition of H_2O_2 to final
concentration of 0.1% preserved the freshness of cows and
buffaloes milk for 12 and 24 hours, respectively at room
temperature for both milks, 0.15% and 0.2% of H_2O_2 were
sufficient to preserve milk for 24 hrs., without showing any
differences in acidity, clot-on-boiling or curdling. (E.L. Safty, M.S.,
Elahmi, M. and Nofal, A.A. in Agricultural Research Review,
1976). Addition of H_2O_2 to milk increased curd tension and
increased the water holding capacity. It was also found that H_2O_2
treated milks were spoiled by proteolytic and sweet curdling
changes while the spoilage of raw milk was due to normal souring.

1. *Bactericidal efficiency of H_2O_2*

Mahmoud, Nagiub and Tanfeek (1984) reported that H_2O_2
was found to be bactericidal to various organisms at variable
rates. The most resistant ones were *Bacillus cereus* spores,
Streptococcus and *Clostriium perfringens* in a descending order.
The most susceptible were the Vegetative cells of aerobic and
anaerobic spore formers as well as *Salmonalla typhimuruim*.
The intermediate were *E. coli*, *Staphylococcus aureus*,
Streptococcus lactis and *S. faecalis*, in this order. It was also found
that the H_2O_2 only temporarily inhibits the growth of some

organisms (e.g. *Streptococcus* spp.) while H_2O_2 has bacteriocidal activity for others (e.g. *E. coli* and *Salmonella typhumurium*). H_2O_2 was also found to be inhibitory to the growth of psychrotrophic bactria. e.g. *pseudomonas* spp. which is helpful in extending storage of refrigerated raw milk.

2. Effect of Concentration

H_2O_2's efficiency as a preservative is found to depend directly on the concentration used, while 0.1-0.2% H_2O_2 has been found to preserve raw milk for 24 hrs. at room temperature. 0.5% H_2O_2 can Preserve raw milk for 48 hrs. at room temperature and for 5-7 days at refrigeration temperature (T. Nassib, H. Abed., 1973).

3. Effect of Temperature

It was found that both total bacterial and colony counts increased during the first day of storage in untreated sample, followed by decrease in their counts after 48 hrs. due to developed acidity (Ewais, Hefnawy and Salam; 1985). The acid development in cow milk was more rapid than buffalo milk in the first 24 hrs. and the reverse was obtained thereafter. In treated samples, both total bacterial and coliform counts continuously decreased with storage and effect of LPS on coliform bacteria was more pronounced in case of buffalo milk where coliform counts was not detected after 48 hrs. in case of 0.1% H_2O_2 treated raw milk and after 24 hrs. in case of 0.2% H_2O_2 treated sample. It was also reported that the acidity and pH of H_2O_2 treated samples were almost unchanged over the storage period of 48 hrs. at room temperature. The concentratio of H_2O_2 used in preservation of milk by LPS at room temperature was found to be inadequate when milk was kept at 35°C. Untreated milk samples failed to keep well for 24 hrs. with rapid proliferation in total bacterial and coliform counts and drop in pH. On the other hand, samples treated with 0.5% H_2O_2 showed great decrease in total bacterial count and coliforms were not detected. The acidity and pH of milk also changed slightly on storage at 35°C. Therefore, at a higher temperature it was found that a much higher H_2O_2 concentration was needed for preservation of raw milk. However, it is advisable to use combined cooling and LPS system using a lower H_2O_2 concentration (0.1%). In this way H_2O_2 used has no deleterious effect on milk constituents and properties, reported on use of high H_2O_2 concentration.

4. Effect on Psychrotrophic Bacteria

Psychrotrophic bacteria do not normally multiply in raw milk held at 5°C during the first 48 hrs. but multiplication will take place if the storage period is prolonged. Both on farms and in dairies it is sometimes desirable to store milk for longer periods, and to do this without producing milk of inferior hygienic quality the multiplication of psychrotrophs need to be prevented. The treatment of milk with H_2O_2 substantially reduces the number of viable organisms during the first few days of storage at refrigeration temperature (Bjorck, 1997) and the milk can thus be stored for up to 5 day without merase in psychrotrophic bacteria. Hadland Sterina (1965) have show that milk product under extremely good hygienic condition can be stored for 4 day without undue bacterial multiplication. The introduce such an hygienic standard on a large scale would however be difficult and would not solve the further increasing strong period at the dairies of milk conaining pschrotrophic organism. The present investigation shows that by activating the LP system by addtion of H_2O_2 it is possible to extend the storage period of refrigerated raw milk inspite of the presence of the psychrotrophic bacteria.

B. FORMALIN TREATMENT

Ibrahim and Amar (1973) reported that the microbial rennet "Rennilase" (MR) as well as calf rennet (CR) were active at pH 5-7 their activity, however, decrease as the pH increased, this being more pronounced with the microbial (MR) then with the CR while when formalin was used as a preservative in a milk, it effected the activity of both enzyme although MR was more effected then CR. At a concentration of 1:500, formalin reduced the activity of MR appreciably and thus it tended to increase the clotting time appreciably.

1. Bactericidal Efficiency of Formalin

Kulshrestha and Marth (1974) reported that formalin was very active against *Escherichia Coli* it caused almost complete inactivation of the organism in less then 2 hrs. when present at a concentration of 1000 ppm.

Formaldehyde even at 100 ppm is quite bactericial and it can reduce the number of organisms to less then 10/ml in less than 11 hrs. the degreee of inactivation increases with time.

In the case of *Salmonella typhimurium* formalin at 1000 ppm inactivated the organisms in less than 2 hrs. and at 100 ppm virtually complete inactivation of the organisms occurs in about 8 hrs. (Kulshrestha, 1974).

Formalin a most detrimental to *Staphylococcus aureus* and at 100 ppm virtually inactivates the organism in less then 2 hrs. Even at 10 ppm formalin is found to significantly inhibit *Staphylococcus aureus*. The degree of inhibition caused by this concentration of formalin greatly increases for 8-11 hrs. of incubation and then decliness.

Formalin is also bactericidal to *Streptococcus lactis*, *Lactobacillus citrovorum* and *Streptococcus thermophilus*. It is reported that formalin at 1000 ppm reduced the population of *Streptococcus* thermophilus by more than 80% in less than 2 hrs. and completely inactivated the organism in 5 hrs. when 100 ppm of formalin was tested, it was always significantly inhibitory to *S. thermophilus* and was most active late in the incubation. At 10 ppm the extent of inhibition was insignificant at the beginning and end of the observation period. A somewhat similar effect was noted with 1 ppm of formalin.

2. Effect of Concentration

Buckley *et al.* (1988) reported that as the concentration of formalin is increased when it is used as a preservative, its efficiency also increases while 0.1% formalin can preserve milk for 2-3 dys. 0.2% formalin can preserve milk for as long as 2 weeks and 0.5% formalin can preserve milk for 28 days at refrigeration temperature.

C. H₂O₂ And Formalin Treatment

Joyce, (1978) reported that phasphotase level in pasteurized liquid milk alter on storage and presence of formaldehyde as preservative negates the phosphatase test, while H_2O_2 was unsuitable as preservative.

Bush and McQueen, (1979) found that formalin in milk decreased the metabolism of all components of milk studied and no volatile fatty acids were produced. Pilkhanem and Bhalerao, (1971) studied the effect of formalin and H_2O_2 on the alkaline phosphatase test in milk. Both formalin and H_2O_2 treated milk sample were preserved at room temperature as well as in the refrigerator. 0.3% treated formalin samples showed a less of 26-28% enzyme activity while H_2O_2 treated milk samples of 0.3% concentration showed a loss of 25-26% enzyme activity. While 0.3% H_2O_2 could preserve milk for 4 days at room temperature and for 11 days at refrigeration temperature. The control milk samples without any preservative were stored for 1 days at room temperature and for 3 days at refrigeration temperature while the enzyme activity lost was about 41% at room temperature and 40% at refrigeration temperature.

These results were in agreement with those of Hahn and Tracy (1938) and Sanders and Sager (1949). These workers have reported a decrease in the enzyme activity of milk samples during storage with the addition of formaldehyde. However, they did not indicate the extent of decrease in the activity. It was also found that formalin treated raw milk samples could be preserved for 28 days at room temperature and 84 days at refrigeration temperature when 0.3% formalin solution was used.

Alf-Laval (1977) reported in the British Patent that although formalin is a much stronger bactericidal agent than H_2O_2 it has not been recommended as an effective milk preservative by the FAO.

The common, local milk vendors still prefer to use formalin as a milk preservative due to their ignorance. Thus the milk that we get at our homes is usually formalin treated.

MATERIAL AND METHOD

A. Collection of Samples

Three sample of raw milk were taken form local milk vendors. The samples were collected in Sterile ground glass stoppered bottles and labelled as sample "A", "B" and "C".

B. Treatment of Samples with Chemicals

Each sample of raw milk was treated with different concentrations of Hydrogen peroxide (H_2O_2) and formalin. Three concentrations of H_2O_2, i.e. 0.1%, 0.1%, 0.2% and 0.5% treated milk samples were prepared and similarly three concentrations of formalin treated milk samples were prepared. Thus, each sample contained six different concentrations of chemically treated milk.

There were 18 milk samples, six samples of milk of sample "A", six of sample "B" and six of sample "C". In addition such each sample contained untreated milk sample to serve as a control.

C. Storage at Room and Refrigeration Temperature

Each sample of milk (chemically treated and untreated) was further divided in two test tubes. The test tubes were cotton plugged and one test tube was kept at room temperature and one at refrigeration temperature. Thus a total of 21 test tubes were stored at room temperature of each sample and 21 test tubes were stored at refrigeration temperature. Careful labelling was done on each test tube to avoid any error or confusion.

D. ·Bacteriological Analysis

Each sample of milk was examined for total bacterial, coliform, and total yeasts and mould coucts. The procedure followed was:

1. Sterlization of Glassware and Equipment

All the glassware like pipettes test-tubes and petri-dishes used in the experiments were throughly cleaned, dried and sterilized in an oven at 160°C for two hrs.

2. *Preparation of Media*

The following media were employed for the enumeration of different organisms.

(a) *Total Bacterial Count*

For general viable count of bacteria a non-selective nutrient medium such as Plate Count Agar also known as Tryptone Glucose Yeast Extract Agar medium was used.

Tryptone	5.0 g
Yeast Extract	2.5 g
Dextrose	1.0 g
Agar	15.0 g
Distilled Water	1 Litre
pH	7.0

The use of nutrient agar is avoided since, it does not allow the growth certain types of bacteria particularly *Streptococci* which may be found quite frequently in food.

For standard plate count the plates were incubated for 48 hrs. at 37°C.

(b) *Total Coliform Count*

Violet Red Bile Agar was used for coliform count.

Yeast Extract	3.0 g
Peptone	7.0 g
Bile Salt (Sodium taurocholate)	1.5 g
NaCl	5.0 g
Lactose	10.0 g
Agar	15.0 g
Neutral red	0.03 g
Crystal violet	0.002 g
Distilled water	1 litre
pH	7.4

MacConkey's Broth and MacConkey's Agar are not satisfactory media for the detection and enumeration of coliform bacteria in milk. Thus viloet Red Bile Agar was used for coliform count.

The plates were incubated at 35°-37°C for 24 hrs for coliform counts. After incubation, the numbers of dark red colonies were counted. Normally typical coliform colonies are 0.5 mm or more in diameter and show evidence of the precipitation of bile salts in the medium immediately surrounding the colonies. Sometimes over crowding of the colonies causes a reduction in size.

(c) Total Yeast and Mould Count

Yeasts and moulds were counted on Potato Dextrose Agar Medium:

Potato	200 g
Dextrose	20 g
Agar-Agar	20 g
Distilled Water	1000 ml
pH	3.5

The pH of the medium was adjusted to 3.5 ± 0.1 by adding 0.17 ml of a sterile 0.1% aqueous solution of tartaric acid for every 10 ml of medium immediately before pouring on plates (American standard methods, 1941).

3. Preparation of Distilled Water

Distilled water was prepared. It was used for serial dilutions of samples of raw milk for the preparation of media.

For serial dilutions sterilized distilled water was used. Distilled water was poured in Erlanmayer flask, cottonplugged and autoclaved for 20 minutes at 15-20 1b/in² for sterilisation.

The prepared media were also sterilised in an autoclave for twenty minutes at 15-20 1b/in² pressure (121°C).

4. Serial Dilution

Each sample of milk was diluted before plating. The dilution were performed with sterlized distilled water. 1 ml of the milk sample was poured into 9 ml of sterilized distilled water to get a dilution of (1:10). One ml of this diluted sample was again transferred into 9 ml of sterilized distilled water to get a dilution of (1:00). This dilution was used for the coliform and yeast and mould count. While a further dilution of 1:1000 was used for total bacterial count or the standard plate count.

5. Pouring the Media and Preparation of Plates

For preparation of plates the pour-plate method was used. Sterilized petridishes were kept inside the laminar air flow. 1 ml of the diluted milk sample was sucked in a pipette and this was then poured into the petri-dish. While transferring the diluted milk sample to the petri-dishes, the end of the pipette was held at an angle of 45° against the petri-dish and the diluted sample was allowed to drain form the graduation mark to the apparent rest point in the tip of the pipette and then touched once against a dry spot on the glass. Care was taken to raise the petri-dish cover only just enough to insert the pipette.

To each of the prepared petrei-plate, the prepared sterilized midium was poured and immediately the medium and inoculum were mixed by shaking the petri-plate in circular movements for 5-10 minutes. Then the medium was allowed to solidify in the petri-dishes. The petri-dishes were then inverted and incubated at an appropriate temperature in the BOD incubator.

6. Plate Counts

After the plates were poured, they were incubated for 4-5 days at 28°C for the yeast and mould count (PDA plates). The Tryptone Dextrose Yeasts Extract Agar medium containing plates were incubated for 48 hours at 37°C for the total bacterial count while the coliforms were counted after an incubation of 24 hours at 37°C (Violete Red Bile agar plates). Further incubation of the coliform plates gave rise to the growth of certain non-coliforms like *Streptococci*, giving inaccurate plate counts.

All results of the plates were counted and average plate counts of the 3 samples (A, B and C) of each chemical treatment (0.1%,

0.2%, 0.5% H_2O_2 and 0.1%, 0.2%, 0.5% formaline and control) of milk calculated and noted down in a tabular form. (Tables 7.1 to 7.6)

7. Pure Culture Isolation

After colony counts, isolation and identification of some colonies was done by the streak-plate technique. A portion of the mixed culture was placed by means of a transfer loop on the surface of an appropriate medium and streaked across the surface by means of a transfer loop. This manipulation "thins out" the bacteria on the agar sugar so that individual bacteria are separated from each other. The streaked plate was incubated at an appropriate temperature for growth of bacteria. This procedure was repeated thrice to get a pure culture of a particular bacteria.

8. Indentification of Bacteria

With the help of a loop, a portoin of the bacterial colony was picked up from the agar surface and placed on a clean slide. A thin smear of the inoculum was prepared and it was then gram stained and observed under a microscope with the help of oil immersion, and then identified.

9. Identification of Yeasts and Moulds

Yeasts and Moulds were identified by staining the yeasts and moulds appearing on the Potato Dextrose Agar plates with cotton blue and observing them under a compound microscope.

RESULT AND DISCUSSION

The changes in total bacterial count, coliform and yeasts and mould counts of untreated, H_2O_2 treated and formalin treated milk sample kept at room temperature are given in Tables 7.1, 7.2 and 7.3 respectively.

The samples which were kept at refrigeration temperature, were examined after 1 day, 2, 4, 7 and 10 days of storage. These samples were periodically plated, incubated and then the number of bacterial, colifrom and yeast and mould colonies counted. The average and range or the total bacterial, coliform and yeasts and mould counts of untreated H_2O_2 treated and formalin treated milk samples (A, B and C) at refrigeration temperature are shown in Tables 7.4, 7.5 and 7.6 respectively.

Beside the colony counts the microscopic examination of some of the pure culture isolated colonies of bacteria was also done. The *Lactobacilli, Streptococci, E. coli, Diplococcus* spp. and rod forms were found to be predominant. Amongst the yeast and moulds species of *Penicillium, Alternaria, Alterraria, Mucor, Phizopus* and a few pink yeasts were found to be predominant.

From the Tables 7.1, 7.2, 7.3, 7.4, 7.5 and 7.6 it is clear that formalin was a better bactericidal chemical than H_2O_2. While the untreated raw milk sample could not be kept for more than 1 day at room temperature. The formalin treated and H_2O_2 treated milk samples could be preserved for 2 days. While 0.1% H_2O_2 could preserve milk for 1 day, 0.2% H_2O_2 , 0.1% and 0.2% formalin treated milk could be kept without spoilage for 2 days. While 0.5% H_2O_2 and 0.5% formalin treated milk could be preserved for 2 days at room temperature.

Similar trend was observed at refigeration temperature when formalin was found to be more bactericidal than H_2O_2. At refrigeration the bacterial count of untreated milk showed a slow increase initially but, after 4 days of storage a rapid increase was seen in the bacterial count. While on H_2O_2 and formalin treatment the bacterial count decreased for the first 4 days and the increases in bacteria after 4 days of storage was found to be less rapid. The milk treated with H_2O_2 and formalin even at 0.1% concentration could preserve milk in good state for 10 days.

The detailed results obtained for different chemical treatment of raw milk are given below :-

I(1) Bacterial Counts at Room Temperature

Untreated milk at room temperature

It was observed that total bacterial count for untreated raw milk increased rapidly on storage at room temperature. Raw milk could not be stored even for 24 hrs. when untreated. The

Table 7.1

Changes in the Bacterial Count (Colony Counts Per ml.) for Three Samples Each of Untreated, H_2O_2 treated and Formalin Treated Raw Milk kept at Room Temperature

Observation (Days of storage)	Treatment Status						
	Control	0.1% H_2O_2	0.2% H_2O_2	0.5% H_2O_2	0.1% Formalin	0.2% Formalin	0.5% Formalin
0	1,77, 000* (163000-196000)	1,59, 666** (142000-178000)	1,37,000** (123000-164000)	91,666** (84000-104000)	1,51,000** (131000-172000)	1,27,000** (114000-147000)	84,000** (76000-98000)
1	2,86,333 (263000-299000)	1,85,333 (174000-196000)	1,29,000 (114000-157000)	71,333 (62000-83000)	1,79,000 (153000-207000)	1,35,333 (127000-151000)	67, 333 (59000-80000)
2	1,77,000 (163000-196000)	3,81,000 (372000-397000)	2,51,000 (239000-268000)	1,51,000 (147000-154000)	4,00,333 (386000-419000)	2,29,000 (216000-100000)	1,20,000 (104000-140000)

*Value for milk prior to addition of chemicals.
**Values, immediately post addition of chemicals.

Table 7.2

Changes in the Colform Count (Colony Counts Per ml.) for Three Samples Each of Untreated, H₂O₂ treated and Formalin Treated Raw Milk kept at Room Temperature

Observation (Days of storage)	Treatmaent Status						
	Control	0.1% H_2O_2	0.2% H_2O_2	0.5% H_2O_2	0.1% Formalin	0.2% Formalin	0.5% Formalin
0	19,666* (18000-20000)	15,866** (13000-18000)	12,866** (10600-15000)	9,233** (7300-11400)	13,900** (11000-16700)	10,333** (8000-12000)	7,100** (6000-8000)
1	33,000 (31000-35000)	12,133 (9800-19000)	9,566 (7000-11800)	6,666 (5000-8000)	10,533 (9000-13000)	3,133 (60 0-9700)	4,133 (3800-4600)
2	25,666 (24000-29000)	9,433 (7500-10800)	5,666 (4000-7000)	3,666 (2400-4300)	7,666 (6600-9600)	4)0 (3400-5900)	2,200 (1600-2500)

*Value for milk prior to addition of chemicals.
**Values, immediately post addition of chemicals.

Table 7.3
Changes in the Yeast and Mould Count (Colony Counts Per ml.) for Three Samples Each of Untreated, H_2O_2 treated and Formalin Treated Raw Milk kept at Room Temperature

Observation (Days of storage)	Treatmaent Status						
	Control	0.1% H_2O_2	0.2% H_2O_2	0.5% H_2O_2	0.1% Formalin	0.2% Formalin	0.5% Formalin
0	8,933* (8000-10000)	7,633** (6500-9000)	5,700** (4500-7000)	3,666** (2000-4000)	7,200** (6000-8600)	5,066** (4000-6200)	2,366** (1500-3000)
1	11,500 (10500-13000)	9,300 (8400-10500)	7,966 (6800-9300)	4,700 (3000-6100)	8,700 (7500-8500)	7,333 (6000-8500)	4,000 (2500-5000)
2	15,333 (13000-18000)	12,266 (11000-14000)	10,000 (9500-11000)	6,900 (4800-8400)	11,266 (10000-12800)	9,366 (8000-10600)	6,066 (4000-7200)

*Value for milk prior to addition of chemicals.
**Values, immediately post addition of chemicals.

Table 7.4

Changes in the total bacterial counts (colony counts per ml.) for three samples each of untreated, H₂O₂ treated and formal in treated raw milk kept at refrigeration temperature.

Observation Days of Storage	Treatment-Status						
	Control	0.1% H₂O₂	0.2% H₂O₂	0.5% H₂O₂	0.1% Formalin	0.2% Formalin	0.5% Formalin
1 Day	1,92,000 (1,63,000-2,21,000)	1,62,000 (1,49,000-1,89,000)	1,37,000 (1,21,000-1,68,000)	1,00,000 (92,000-1,12,000)	1,52,000 (1,38,000-1,77,000)	1,24,000 (1,02,000-1,52,000)	88,000 (81,500-1,01,000)
2 Day	2,19,000 (1,82,000-2,52,000)	1,38,666 (1,21,000-1,62,000)	1,18,000 (1,01,000-1,44,000)	85,666 (78,000-98,000)	1,30,333 (1,19,000-1,51,000)	1,02,000 (84,000-1,30,000)	74,333 (68,000-84,000)
4 Day	2,64,333 (2,48,000-2,93,000)	1,05,666 (1,00,000-1,16,000)	90,333 (8,000-1,02,000)	61,000 (57,000-57,000)	93,000 (87,000-1,04,000)	77,333 (71,000-82,000)	47,000 (42,600-53,000)
7 Day	3,17,000 (3,09,000-3,42,000)	1,28,333 (1,23,000-1,32,000)	1,10,666 (1,01,000-1,12,000)	78,666 (73,000-89,000)	1,12,000 (1,01,000-1,26,000)	94,666 (89,000-98,000)	65,666 (61,000-69,000)
10 Day	5,19,333 (5,02,000-5,30,000)	1,78,333 (1,70,000-1,89,000)	1,49,333 (1,39,000-1,61,000)	1,15,000 (1,07,000-1,24,000)	1,52,333 (1,38,000-1,73,000)	1,24,000 (1,06,000-1,45,000)	88,000 (80,000-93,000)

* Value for raw milk prior to addition of chemicals in raw milk = 1,77,000 Colonies/Ml.

Table 7.5

Changes in the total coliform counts (colony counts per ml.) for three samples each of untreated, H_2O_2 treated and formal in treated raw milk kept at refrigeration temperature.

Time of Storage / Days of Storage	Treatment-Status						
	Control	0.1% H_2O_2	0.2% H_2O_2	0.5% H_2O_2	0.1% Formal in	0.2% Formal in	0.5% Formal in
1 Day	22,500 (21,000-24,000)	18,000 (16,000-21,000)	14,733 (12,800-17,000)	11,333 (9,000-14,000)	16,566 (15,000-19,000)	13,366 (11,000-16,000)	10,300 (2,500-11,800)
2 Day	25,000 (23,000-27,000)	14,866 (12,900-17,000)	12,300 (10,300-14,000)	9,300 (7,600-12,000)	12,900 (12,100-14,800)	11,066 (8,800-13,400)	8,266 (7,000-9,000)
4 Day	28,333 (26,000-31,000)	11,200 (9,600-13,000)	9,400 (7,900-11,000)	6,966 (6,000-8,600)	9,600 (8,000-9,200)	8,533 (71,000-9,600)	6,433 (5,600-7,000)
7 Day	25,433 (23,600-28,000)	8,433 (7,400-9,500)	7,633 (6,100-9,600)	4,700 (3,900-5,800)	7,400 (7,000-8,000)	6,200 (5,800-6,700)	3,866 (3,800-4,000)
10 Day	22,666 (21,000-25,000)	6,500 (5,300-8,000)	5,600 (4,200-7,000)	1,966 (1,700-2,200)	5,333 (5,000-6,000)	4,866 (3,600-4,100)	1,500 (1,100-1,800)

* Value for raw milk prior to addition of chemicals in raw milk = 19,666 Colonies/Ml.

Table 7.6

Changes in the total bacterial counts (colony counts per ml.) for three samples each of untreated, H₂O₂ treated and formal in treated raw milk kept at refrigeration temperature.

Time of Storage	Treatment-Status						
Days of Storage	Control	0.1% H₂O₂	0.2% H₂O₂	0.5% H₂O₂	0.1% Formal in	0.2% Formal in	0.5% Formal in
1 Day	10,233	8,166	6,966	4,993	7,766	6,533	4,533
	(9,700-11,000)	(7,000-9,500)	(5,900-8,000)	(4,200-5,500)	(6,700-9,000)	(5,300-7,500)	(4,000-5,000)
2 Day	9,100	7,333	5,766	3,933	6,866	5,566	3,500
	(8,400-10,200)	(6,300-9,000)	(5,000-6,500)	(3,400-4,400)	(5,900-8,000)	(4,500-6,200)	(3,200-4,000)
4 Day	7,533	6,066	4,066	2,733	5,366	4,333	2,266
	(7,100-8,300)	(5,000-7,600)	(3,900-4,000)	(2,500-3,000)	(4,700-6,200)	(3,300-5,000)	(2,000-2,500)
7 Day	6,133	4,700	2,766	1,500	4,000	2,300	1,133
	(5,600-7,000)	(3,600-6,300)	(2,600-2,900)	(1,200-1,700)	(3,300-4,600)	(2,000-2,500)	(1,000-1,200)
10 Day	4,600	3,333	1,533	800	2,500	1,100	500
	(4,000-5,800)	(2,100-5,000)	(1,400-1,700)	(600-900)	(2,000-3,000)	(1,000-1,200)	(100-600)

* Value for raw milk prior to addition of chemicals in raw milk = 8,933 Colonies/Ml.

changes in untreated raw milk kept at room temperature were found to be:

(i)   On 1 day of storage there was an increase of 61.7% in the total bacterial count.

(ii) On 2 days of storage there was an increase of 219.4% in the total bacterial count with respect to the initial bacterial count and an increase of 97.4% with respect to 1st day's bacterial count.

The milk was completely co-agulated/curdled by the 2nd day of storage.

0.1% H_2O_2 treatment at room temperature

When this milk sample was treated with 0.1% H_2O_2 the raw milk could be preserved for 1 day without spoilage when kept at room temperature. The percentage changes in 0.1% H_2O_2 treated raw milk kept at room temperature were as follows:

(i)   As soon as 0.1% H_2O_2 was added to milk (fresh raw milk – 0 day) there was a 9.8% decrease in the bacterial count as compared to the untreated sample.

(ii) On 24 hours of storage there was in increase of 16.07% in the bacterial count as compared to an increase of 61.7% in the ease of untreated raw milk samples after 24 hours of storage. Thus there was decrease of 35.3% with respect to the untreated 1 day raw milk sample. While there was only an increase of 4.7% in the bacterial count of 0.1% H_2O_2 1-day sample when compared with the untreated 0-day sample.

(iii) On 2 days of storage there was an increase of 138.6% in the total bacterial count with respect to initial bacterial count and an increase of 115.2% when compared with the intitial bacterial count of untreated 0-day sample. The increase in bacterial count was very rapid after 2 days of storage as compared to 24 hours of storage. 105.5% increase in bacterial count was observed as compared to the 1st day 0.1% H_2O_2 treated bacterial count.

Thus, it was observed that with 0.1% H_2O_2 milk could be stored for 24 hors without spoilage but after 24 hours this concentration of H_2O_2 could not prove to be bactericidal and a very rapid increase in bacterial count was observed. The raw milk treated with 0.1% H_2O_2 did not curdle after 24 hours of storage, while on 48 hours of storage sweet curdling of raw milk (including spoilage of milk) was observed.

0.2% H_2O_2 treatment at room temperature

When the raw milk sample was treated with 0.2% H_2O_2 the milk could be preserved for 1 day without spoilage at room temperature. While the milk did not show co-agulation curdling after 48 hours of storage at room temperature, but there was an increase in the bacterial count which were well above the standard consumable bacterial count (i.e. 1.0-2.0 × 10^5 ml^{-1}. International Dairy Federation, 1974). The percentage change in 0.2% H_2O_2 treatment raw milk kept at room temperature were as follows:

(i)   As soon as 0.2% H_2O_2 was added to fresh raw milk there was a 22.5% decrease in the bacterial count as compared to the untreated sample while there was only 9.8% decrease when treated with 0.1% H_2O_2.

(ii) On 24 hours of storage there was a decrease of 5.8% in bacterial count as compared to the 0-day of 0.2% H_2O_2 treated sample and a decrease of 27.1% with respect to untreated 0-day sample. While there was an increase of 16.07% in the case of 0.1% H_2O_2 treated sample on storage for 24 hours.

(iii) After 48 hours of storage there was an increase of 83.4% with respect to the 0-day treated sample and an increase of 94.8% with respect to 24 hours treated sample. Thus, the increase was less rapid as compared to an increase of 138.6% of 0.1% H_2O_2 treated sample stored for 48 hours.

There was an increase of only 41.9% with respect to the untreated 0-day sample while in the case of 0.1% H_2O_2 treated raw milk there was an increase of 115.2% after 48 hours of storage.

There was a 32.6% decrease in the bacterial count of raw milk treated with 0.1 H_2O_2 after 48 hours of storage as compared to 2nd day bacterial count of untreated sample. While in the case of 0.2% H_2O_2 treatment there was decrease of 55.5%. Thus, after 48 hours of storage 0.2% H_2O_2 treated milk sample contained about half the microflora as compared to that of the untreated 48 hours stored sample.

0.5% H_2O_2 treatment at room temperature

When the milk sample was treated with 0.5% milk could be stored at room temperature without spoilage for 48 hours. There was a rapid decrease in the bacterial count for the first 24 hours but later an increase in the bacterial count was observed. The percentage change in the bacterial count of 0.5% H_2O_2 treated raw milk samples were as follows :

(i)   On addition of 0.5% H_2O_2 to fresh raw milk there was a 48.2% decrease in bacterial count as compared to the untreated sample. Thus, about half the bacteria were destroyed on addition of 0.5% H_2O_2.

(ii) After 24 hours of storage a further 22.18% decrease in bacterial count was observed which amount to a decrease of 59.7% with respect to the fresh untreated raw milk sample. This bacterial count was 75% less than the vales obtained after 24 hours of storage of the untreatment raw milk sample. Thus, it was found that after 24 hours of storage only 25% bacteria were present in raw milk treated with 0.5% H_2O_2, as compared to the value obtained after 24 hours of storage of untreated raw milk.

(iii) On 2 days of storage there was an increase of 111.7% with respect to 1 day 0.5% H_2O_2 treated sample which amounted an increase of 64.7% with respect to the 0-day, 0.5% H_2O_2 treated sample. While an increase of 83.4 was observed o storage of 0.2% H_2O_2 treated milk for 2 days.

When compared with the bacterial count of fresh raw milk sample (0-day untreated) there was a 15.2% decrease in bacterial count after 48 hrs. of storage of 0.5% H_2O_2 treated sample. This amounted to 73.3% decrease with respect to the bacterial count of 2 day stored untreated sample. Thus, (as observed after 24 hrs of storage) there was still a decrease of 3/4th of the bacteria (i.e. ¼th of the bacteria were present) in 0.5% H_2O_2 treated sample after 48 hrs. of storage as compared to that of untreated raw milk stored for 48 hours.

Even after 2 days of storage at room temperature raw milk treated with 0.5% H_2O_2 could be preserved without spoilage.

0.1% Formalin treatment at room temperature

When raw milk was treated with 0.1% formalin, it showed a similar bactericidal activity as that observed after treatment with 0.1% H_2O_2, but its efficiency was much more than that of H_2O_2.

(i) As soon as 0.1% formalin was added there was a 14.7% decrease in the bacterial count as compared to the untreated sample while in the case of 0.1% H_2O_2 there was only a decrease of 9.8%.

(ii) On 24 hrs. of storage there was a 18.7% increase in the bacterial count with respect to 0-day 1% formalin treated sample while in the case of 0.1% H_2O_2 an increase of 16.07% was observed. Thus, after 24 hrs. of storage both H_2O_2 and formalin were almost equally efficient against bacteria. Due to formalin's stronger bactericidal efficiency, it brought about an increase of only 1.32% with respect to the untreated raw milk (0-day). While an increase of 4.7% was observed in the case of 0.1% H_2O_2 treated raw milk with respect to the untreated raw milk (0-day).

(iii) After 2 days of storage a much rapid increase in bacterial count was observed as compared to the H_2O_2 treated raw milk. Thus it was found that while formalin in a stronger bactericide than H_2O_2 but it looses its efficiency after a few hours; while H_2O_2 does not loose its bactericidal property fast.

On 2 days of storage 165.12% increase in bacterial count was observed in 0.1% formalin treated sample and an increase of 138.6% was observed in 0.1% H_2O_2 treated sample when compared to the initial bacterial count, and an increase of 126.2% with respect to 0-day treated sample for 0.1% formalin treated milk, while, for 0.1% H_2O_2 treated sample an increase of 115.2% was observed.

0.2% formlain treatment at room tempeature

0.2% formalin treated milk could be stored at room temperature for 48 hrs. without any spoilage, but due to it's rapid increase in bacterial count after 48 hrs. of storage it was not hygienically recommended for drinking purpose after 48 hours:

(i) As soon as 0.2% formalin was added to fresh milk there was a 28.6% decrease (22.5% for 0.2%, H_2O_2) in the bacterial count as compared to the untreated sample.

(ii) On 24 hrs. of storage there was a decrease of 6.28% as compared to the 0-day 0.2% formalin treated sample and a decrease of 23.6% with respect to untreated 0-day sample while in the case of 0.2% H_2O_2 the decrease was 27.1%. Thus, there was 5.9% increase with respect to one day 0.2% H_2O_2 treated sample.

(iii) After 24 hrs of storage there was an increase of 79.8% with respect to the 0-day formalin treated sample and an increase of 69.2% with respect to 24 hrs treated sample. Thus, the increase was less rapid as compared to that obtained for 0.2% H_2O_2 treatment. There was a 8.7% decrease with respect to 2-day 0.2% H_2O_2 treated sample. There was an increase of 22.6% (41.9% for 0.2% H_2O_2) with respect to the untreated 0-day sample.

0.5% Formalin treatment at room temperature

When raw milk was treated with 0.5% formalin it could be stored at room temperature for 48 hrs. without spoilage. Infect, even after 48 hrs. the bacterial count was much below the initial bacterial count of fresh raw milk. On the 1st day a decrease in bacterial count was observed, showing that 0.5% formalin was exhibiting bactericidal property up to 24 hrs. but after 24 hrs. there was an increase in the bacterial count. Though even after 2 days the count was much below the initial bacterial count:

(i)   On addition of 0.5% formalin to fresh raw milk there was a 52.5% decrease in bacterial count (48.2% decrease for 0.5% H_2O_2) as compared to the untreated sample.

(ii) After 24 hrs. of storage a further 19.8% decrease in bacterial count was observed which amounted to a decrease of 61.9% with respect to the fresh untreated raw milk sample. This bacterial count was 76.4% less than that obtained after 24 hrs. of storage of the untreated raw milk sample.

(iii) On 2-day of storage there was an increase of 78.2% with respect to 1 day 0.5% formalin treated sample which amounted to an increase of 40.4% with respect to the 0-day 0.5% formalin treated sample. While an increase of 64.7% was observed on 48 hrs. of storage of 0.5% H_2O_2 treated milk at room temperature.

When compared with the bacterial count of fresh raw milk (0-day untreated) there was a 32.2% decrease (15.2% decrease with 0.5% H_2O_2) in bacterial count after 48 hrs. of storage of 0.5% formalin treated sample. This amounted to a 78.7% decrease with respect to the bacterial count of 2 days stored untreated sample (73.3% decrease for 0.5% H_2O_2).

Thus, even after 48 hrs of storage 0.5% formalin treated milk contained 2/3rd of the bacterial that were present in the fresh untreated raw milk.

The above discussion clearly indicated that as the concentration of chemicals increased so did the duration of milk preservation. Formalin was found to be a stronger preservative as compared to H_2O_2 at room temperature.

A similar trend was also found for the coliform and yeast and mould count for different chemical treatment at room temperature.

(2) Coliform counts at room temperature

Untreated milk

An increase in colifrm count was observed after 24 hours of storage but due to increased acidity the count decreased after 48 hours.

Chemical treated milk

On treatment with H_2O_2 and formalin there was a steady decrease in coliform counts for both 24 hrs. and 48 hrs. of storage of milk. Formalin was found to be a better bactericide against coliforms as compared to H_2O_2.

(3) Yeast and Mould Counts at Room Temperature

Untreated milk

In untreated milk samples a steady increase in yeast and mould counts were observed as the time of storage increased.

Chemically treated milk

On treatment with H_2O_2 and formalin there was a decrease in yeast and mould count when the chemical was added but after storage for 24-48 hrs. the yeast and mould count was found to increase. Thus, it was found that both these chemicals could prove to be fungicidal when added to milk but could not restrict yeast and mould growth for long period of milk storage (i.e. 24-48 hours).

II. REFRIGERATION TEMPERATURE PRESERVATION OF MILK

(1) Bacterial Counts At Refrigeration Temperature

Untreated raw milk

When untreated raw milk was stored at refrigeration temperature there was an increase in bacterial count. The increase was slow for the first two days but after two days of storage rapid increase in bacterial count was observed due to the growth of psychrotrophic bacteria. The percentage changes observed in untreated raw milk kept at refrigeration temperature were as follows :

(i)   After 1 day of storage 8.4% increase in bacterial count took place.

(ii) After 2 days of storage there was an increase of 27.1% with respect to the initial sample that amounted to 14.4% increase with respect to the bacterial count obtained after 24 hours of storage.

(iii) After 4 days of storage there was 49.3% increase in bacterial count which amounted to 20.3% increase with respect to 48 hrs. stored raw milk.

(iv) After 7 days of storage there was a 79.09% increase in bacterial count which meant a 19.9% increase with respect to 4 days stored sample.

(v) After 10 days of storage there was a 193.4% increase in bacterial count which amounted to a 63.8% increase with respect to 7 days stored sample. Thus there was a rapid increase in bacterial count after the 7th day of storage.

Thus, untreated raw milk could be preserved at refrigeration temperature for 2 days in a hygienically good state. Although milk did not show curdling even after 7 days of storage but due to high bacterial count this milk was not hygienically consumable.

(vi) When the milk was treated with H_2O_2 or formalin the number of viable organisms substantially reduced during the first 4 days of storage but an increase was observed after 4 days of storage.

0.1% H_2O_2 and 0.1% formalin treatment

0.1% formalin was found to be a better preservative then 0.1% H_2O_2. The following percentage change in bacterical counts were observed for 0.1% formalin and 0.1% H_2O_2 treated raw milk stored at referigeration temperature.

(i) On 24 hours of storage there was a 1.8% inçrease in bacterial count of 0.1% H_2O_2 treated sample, while formilin treated sample exhibited a 0.88% increase only. When compared with the bacterial count of 0 day untreated sample (fresh raw milk) 0.1% H_2O_2 treated sample showed a 8.09% decrease while 0.1% formalin treated sample showed a 13.9% decrease.

(ii) After 2 days of storage there was a further decrease of 14.7% for 0.1% H_2O_2 treated sample and 14.4% for 0.1% formalin treated sample which meant a 13.7% decrease for 0.1% H_2O_2 and 15.8% decrease for 0.1% formalin treated milk with respect to the initial 0.1% treated samples of H_2O_2 and formalin respectively.

When compared with the bacterial count of fresh raw milk there was a 21.6% decrease and 26.3% decrease for 0.1% H_2O_2 and 0.1% formalin treatment respectively.

(iii) After 4 days storage there was a further decrease of 23.7% for 0.1% H_2O_2 and 28.6% for 0.1% formalin treated sample which amounted to a total 33.8%   and 38.4% decrease in bacterial count for 0.1% H_2O_2 and 0.1% formalin treated samples respectively when compared to the 0-day treated sample.

With respect to the bacterial count of fresh raw milk there was a 40.3% and 47.4% decrease for 0.1% H_2O_2 and 0.1% formalin treated samples respectively.

(iv) The bacterial count after 7 days of storage showed a 21.4% and 20.4% increase for 0.1% H_2O_2 and 0.1% formalin treated samples respectively with respect to the bacterial count of 4 days stored samples. This there was a 19.6% decrease for 0.1% H_2O_2 and 25.8% decrease for 0.1% formalin treated samples as compared to the fresh treated milk samples.

There was a 27.5% and 36.7% decrease for 0.1% H_2O_2 and 0.1% formalin treated samples respectively, as comapred to the counts of fresh untreated raw milk.

(v) On 10 days of storage there was a further increase of 38.9% for 0.1% H_2O_2 and 36.01% for 0.1% formalin treated samples which amounted to 11.7% increase for 0.1% H_2O_2 treated and only 0.88% increase for 0.1% formalin treated samples when comapred with the fresh treated milk samples.

Thus, 0.1% H_2O_2 treated samples showed a 0.75% increase and 0.1% formalin treated samples showed a 14.12% decrease in bacterial count as compared to the counts of fresh untreated raw milk.

Thus, 0.1% H_2O_2 and 0.1% formalin treatment count preserve raw milk for as long as 10 days without a significant increase in a bacterial count. The milk so preserved was of hygencally good quality. Thus, even such a small concentration of H_2O_2 or formalin was enough for milk preservation for long periods at refrigeration temperature, while the same concentration of H_2O_2 and formalin count not preserve milk for more than 1 days at room temperature. It can thus be concluded that both H_2O_2 and formalin are very effective against psychrotrophic bacteria in milk.

0.2% H_2O_2 and 0.2% formalin treatment

Although 0.1% H_2O_2 and 0.1% formalin treatment was found to be sufficient for long time preservation of milk at refrigeration tempreature, still observations for 0.2% and 0.5% H_2O_2 and formalin treated milk samples were taken. Since these observations were not significant form the practical application point of view they have been shown in a sample tabular form. (Table 7.7).

Table 7.7 clearly indicates the greater bactericidal property of 0.2% formalin treated milk sample, as compared to 0.2% H_2O_2 treated milk sample and a similar effect was also seen with 0.5% H_2O_2 and formalin treated milk samples.

0.5% H_2O_2 and 0.5%formalin treatment

The percentage changes is bacterial count at refrigeration temperature for 0.5% H_2O_2 and 0.5% formalin treated milk samples are shown in Table 7.8.

(2) Coliform Counts at Refrigeration Temperature

Untreated milk

There was an increase in coliform count of untreated raw milk when stored at refrigeration temperature for up to 4 days. Due to increasing acidity and increase in psychrotrophic bacteria, the coliform count decreases by the 7th day of storage at refrigeration temperature.

Chemically treated milk

H_2O_2 and formalin treated milk samples show a steady

TABLE 7.7

Days of Storage	Percentage change with respect to fresh untreated milk sample (0-Day)		Percentage change with respect to fresh treated milk sample (0-Day)		Percentage change with respect to fresh previous days count (0-Day)	
	0.2% H_2O_2	0.2 Formalin	0.2% H_2O_2	0.2% Formalin	0.2% H_2O_2	0.2% Formalin
01 Day	(-)22.4%	(-)29.9%	(+)24%	(-)2.6%	(+)24%	(-)2.6%
02 Days	(-)33.3%	(-)42.3%	(-)13.8%	(-)19.8%	(-)14.07%	(-)17.7%
04 Days	(-)48.9%	(-)56.3%	(-)34.06%	(-)39.2%	(-)23.4%	(-)24.2%
07 Days	(-)37.4%	(-)46.5%	(-)19.2%	(-)25.6%	(+)22.5%	(+)22.4%
10 Days	(-)15.6%	(-)29.9%	(+)9.002%	(-)2.6%	(+)34.9%	(+)30.9%

(+) : Increase in Bacterial count.
(-) : Decrease in Bacterial count.

TABLE 7.8

Days of Storage	Percentage change with respect to fresh untreated milk sample (0-Day)		Percentage change with respect to fresh treated milk sample (0-Day)		Percentage change with respect to fresh previous days count (0-Day)	
	0.5% H_2O_2	0.5 Formalin	0.5% H_2O_2	0.5% Formalin	0.5% H_2O_2	0.5% Formalin
01 Day	(-) 43.5%	(-) 49.9%	(+) 9.09%	(+) 5.5%	(+) 9.09%	(+) 5.5%
02 Days	(-) 51.6%	(-) 58.0%	(-) 6.5%	(-) 11.5%	(-) 14.3%	(-) 16.2%
04 Days	(-) 65.5%	(-) 73.4%	(-) 73.4%	(-) 44.04%	(-) 28.8%	(-) 36.7%
07 Days	(-) 55.5%	(-) 62.9%	(-) 14.18%	(-) 21.8%	(+) 28.9%	(+) 39.7%
10 Days	(-) 35.02%	(-) 50.28%	(+) 25.4%	(+) 4.7%	(+) 45.18%	(+) 34.01%

(+) : Increase in Bacterial count.
(-) : Decrease in Bacterial count.

decrease in coliform counts on storage at refrigeration temperature. The same trend in coliform counts was also observed for milk stored at room temperature. Formalin was found to be a stronger bactericide then H_2O_2.

(3) Yeast and Mould Counts At Refrigeration Temperature

Untreated milk

In untreated milk samples a steady decrease in yeast and mould counts were observed as the time of storage increased at refrigeration temperature.

Chemically treated milk

On treatment with H_2O_2 and formalin there was a decrease in yeast and mould count on storage at refrigeration temperature. About 91% of yeast and mould were detroyed by 0.5% H_2O_2 and 94.4% decrease was observed for 0.5% formalin treated milk samples stored for 10 days at refrigeration temperature.

Thus, it was finally concluded that formalin was a better preservative than H_2O_2, but H_2O_2 has been recommended as one of the best chemical treatments that could be safely uses to prevent the spoilage of milk for human consumption by the FAO meeting of Experts (1957).

The study done showed that for room temperature storage of raw milk 0.1% H_2O_2 and formalin could preserve raw milk for one day. 0.2% formalin could preserve raw milk for 2 days but 0.2% H_2O_2 was not sufficient to preserve raw milk for 2 days. While 0.5% H_2O_2 and 0.5% formalin could preserve raw milk at room temperature 2 days in hygiencially good quality.

While 0.1% H_2O_2 and 0.1% formalin was found to preserve raw milk for upto 10 days at refrigeration temperature. Thus, the efficiency of chemicals as preservatives, was found to increase as the temperature of storage decreased. A combined treatment of cooling and treatment of small concentration of H_2O_2 formalin can be used for long term preservation of milk (raw milk).

Summary

Prevention of raw milk souring during storage and for transportation can help to improve and enhance increased milk production and utilization. In most developed, countries the combination of usually poor hygience standards, high ambient temperature and lack of refrigeration facilities render milk very much susceptible to spoilage due to common lactic acid bacteria. Growth of psychrotrophic bacteria during prolonged refrigerated storage raw milk poses additional problems as such organisms can produce heat resistant proteolytic and lipolytic enzymes responsible for undesirable changes in milk products.

As we make changes in the production, processing, and distribution of milk and milk products, we solve some problems and apparently create new difficulties. Modern dairy farms have highly mechanised milking systems together with on-farm regrigerated bulk storage tanks, and these innovations seem to have changed the quality of raw milk by altering its microflora. The shift in kinds of micro-organisms has been in favour of psychrotrophic bacteria. These psychrotrophic bacteria are responsible for causing poor flavours in milk. We have known for many years that some micro-organisms can multiply in cold milk, but for a long time, the milk industry got along reasonably well by obeying the cardinal rules of keeping milk and cold. However, with the introduction of bulk handling, along with refrigerated milk storage, defects in milk quality began showing up in different milk marketing areas.

Suitable chemical preservations mathod(s) can offer immediate and practical solution to these current problems. As all micro-organisms do not react alike when exposed to chemical biocides or disinfectants, the eradication of micro-organisms by chemical methods can be a complex undertaking and even a so-called "Over-Kill" which may be thought of as using excessive amounts of chemicals to destroy, bacteria may prove unsatisfactory.

Although formalin which is a liquid and has to erroneous results when testing milk for protein content, has never been used or recommended as an effective milk preservative, but it has been used as a traditional preservative by local milk vendors of our country. While Siegenthaler (1965) reported that H_2O_2 treatment of milk could preserve milk in hygienically good state.

The purpose of present study was to provide some preliminary date on the effectiveness of different concenterations of H_2O_2 and formalin in the preservation of raw milk at both room and refrigeration temperature.

1. It was found that bacterial count at room temperature for untreated raw milk increased rapidly on storage at room temperature. The milk showed curdling coagulation within 24 hrs. of storage.
   On treatment with 0.1% H_2O_2 /0.1% formalin treated milk could be preserved for 24 hrs. without spoilage but curdling/co-agulation (Spoilage) occurred after 48 hrs. of storage.
   0.2% H_2O_2 /0.2% formalin treated milk could be preserved for 24 hrs. in good hygienic state, although no curdling/co-agulation of milk took place after 48 hrs of storage but 0.2% H_2O_2 treated milk showed bacterial count much above the standard consumable bacterial count. While 0.2% formalin could be preserved without spoilage even after 48 hrs. of storage. 0.5% H_2O_2 /0.5% formalin treated milk could be preserved for 48 hrs. without spoilage at room temperature.

2. Coliform counts increased during the first 24 hrs. of storage in untreated milk samples but due to increased acidity coliform counts decreased during the 2nd day of storage. While for treated milk there was a steady decrease in bacterial count as the storage period was increased.

3. In untreated milk samples an increase in yeast and mould counts were observed as the time of storage increased. On treatment with H_2O_2 /formalin there was a decrease in yeast and mould count when the chemical was added but after storage for 24-48 hours the yeast and mould count was found to increase.

4. The bacterial count for untreated raw milk stored at refrigeration temperature shows a slow increase in bacterial count for the first 48 hrs but after 48 hrs of storage a rapid increase in bacterial count is observed

due to the growth of psychrotrophic bacteria. The milk can be stored for two days without spoilage. Though no curdling/co-agulation of milk occurs but due to high bacterial count milk is not consumable after 48 hrs. of storage.

0.1% H_2O_2 /0.1% formalin treated milk was found to preserve milk up to 10 days wifhout spoilage. There was a decrease in bacterial count during the first 4 days of storage but later an increase in bacteria count was observed.

0.2% H_2O_2/formalin and 0.5% H_2O_2 /formalin treated milk was also found to show a decrease in bacterial count during the first four days of storage but later an increase in bacterial count was observed.

5. Coliform counts increased in untreated raw milk when stored at refrigeration temperature upto 4 days. Due to increasing acidity and increase in psychrotorpic bacteria, the coliform count decreases by the 7th day of storage refrigeration temperature.

    While H_2O_2 and formalin treated milk samples show a steady decrease in coliform counts on storage at refrigeration temperature. The same trend in coliform counts was also observed for milk stored a room temperature.

6. In untreated milk samples a steady decrease in yeast and mould counts was observed as the time of storage increased at refrigeration temperature.

    On treatment with H_2O_2 /formalin there was a decrease in yeast and mould count on storage at regrigeration temperature.

7. the organisms isolated from different samples of milk were characterized and identified as:

    (a) *Bacteria*: Species of *Lactobacillus, Streptococous, Micrococcus, Diplococcus,* and *Bacillus* were observed.

    (b) *Coliforms: Escherichia coli, Aerobacter aerogenes*

    (c) *Yeasts*: Few pink yeasts probably belonging to *Rhodotorulaceae.*

    (d) *Moulds*: Species of *Penicillium, Cladosporium, Alternaria, Mucor, Rizopus* and *Fusarium.*

Milk preservatives, some of which were sold under trade names, were at one time rather widely used, but regulations prohibiting the practive have largely eliminated it. The present availability of ice and refrigerating machinery provides adequate facilities for holding milk so there is no longer need to use preservatives, except in samples intended for special purposes.

In a developing country, like India refrigeration facilities are not available to poor local milk vendors. Due to the tropical climatic conditions (favouring growth of mesophilic and thermophilic bacteria), milk is usually spiled during transportation or storage. Even in countries where refrigeration facilities are available. Milk slowly degrades in its quality due to growth of psychrotrophic bacteria. Both these factors make the use of chemical preservatives "a necessary evil" for storage and preservation of milk.

However, with combined use of refrigeration and chemicals (in small concentrations) milk can be stored/preserved in a hygienically consumable state. From the study done on the effect of hydrogen peroxide and formalin on the microflora of milk at room and refrigeration temperature, it was found that:

— 0.1% H_2O_2/0.1% formalin could preserve milk (raw) for 24 hrs without spoilage.

THE CHEMICAL AND MICROBIOLOGICAL ANALYSIS OF SAMPLES OF KHOA BASED SWEETS COLLECTED FROM LOCAL MARKET

Abbreviations

B	=	Burfi
P	=	Peda
L	=	Lodge
Sc	=	Sweets kept in show cases
OP	=	Sweet kept in open pan
SPC	=	Standard Plate Count
SC	=	Spore Count
YMC	=	Yeast and mould Count
Coli	=	Coliform Count

SAMPLE NO. –1 B/SC

Chemical Analysis

1.	Moisture	8.10
2.	Fat	17.00
3.	Ash	3.2
4.	Sugar	50.92 (18.6 ml)
	(*Bura*)	56.57
5.	Protein	20.78

Microbiological Analysis

1.	S.P.C.	3×10^4
2.	S.P.	7×10^3
3.	Coli	No Colony
4.	Y.M.C.	No Colony
5.	Pathogens	5×10^2

SAMPLE NO. – 2   B/SC
Chemical Analysis

1.	Moisture	11.20
2.	Fat	18.20
3.	Ash	3.4
4.	Sugar	43.42 (22.0 ml)
	(*Bura*)	48.13
5.	Protein	23.78

Microbiological   Analysis

1.	SPC	4×10^4
2.	SP	15.5×10^3
3.	Coli	No Colony
4.	YMC	No Colony
5.	Pathogens	5.5×10^2

SAMPLE NO. – 3   B/OP
Chemical   Analysis

1.	Moisture	12.60
2.	Fat	21.00
3.	Ash	4.5
4.	Sugar	33.44 (28.2 ml)
	(*Bura*)	37.15
5.	Protein	28.46

Microbiological   Analysis

1.	SPC	13.5×10^4
2.	SC	41.5×10^3
3.	Coli	No Colony
4.	YMC	No Colony
5.	Pathogens	10.5×10^2

SAMPLE NO. – 4   B/SC
Chemical   Analysis

1.	Moisture	14.00
2.	Fat	16.20
3.	Ash	3.7
4.	Sugar	49.40 (19.2 ml)
	(*Bura*)	54.88
5.	Protein	16.70

Microbiological   Analysis

1. SPC 2×10^4
2. SP 32.5×10^3
3. Coli   No Colony
4. YMC   No Colony
5. Pathogens 4×10^2

SAMPLE NO. – 5   B/SC
Chemical Analysis

1. Moisture   10.50
2. Fat   17.20
3. Ash   2.5
4. Sugar   32.68 (28.6 ml)
      (*Bura*)   36.31
5. Protein   37.12

Microbiological Analysis

1. SPC 11×10^4
2. SC 30×10^3
3. Coli   No Colony
4. YMC   No Colony
5. Pathogens 6.5×10^2

SAMPLE NO. – 6   B/SC
Chemical Analysis

1. Moisture   13.40
2. Fat   19.40
3. Ash   2.8
4. Sugar   37.24 (25.4 ml)
      (*Bura*)   41.37
5. Protein   27.16

Microbiological Analysis

1. SPC 3.5×10^4
2. SC 20×10^3
3. Coli   No Colony
4. YMC   No Colony
5. Pathogens 4.5×10^2

SAMPLE NO. – 7   B/OP
Chemical Analysis

1.	Moisture	13.20
2.	Fat	18.00
3.	Ash	1.2
4.	Sugar	50.92 (18.6 ml)
	(*Bura*)	56.57
5.	Protein	16.68

Microbiological Analysis

1.	SPC	8×10^4
2.	SC	13×10^3
3.	Coli	No Colony
4.	YMC	No Colony
5.	Pathogens	3×10^2

SAMPLE NO. – 8   B/SC
Chemical Analysis

1.	Moisture	11.25
2.	Fat	21.20
3.	Ash	1.4
4.	Sugar	44.84 (21.2 ml)
	(*Bura*)	49.82
5.	Protein	21.31

Microbiological Analysis

1.	SPC	5.5×10^4
2.	SC	12×10^3
3.	Coli	No Colony
4.	YMC	No Colony
5.	Pathogens	9×10^2

SAMPLE NO. – 9   B/SC
Chemical Analysis

1.	Moisture	14.30
2.	Fat	16.80
3.	Ash	1.5
4.	Sugar	58.52 (16.2 ml)
	(*Bura*)	65.02
5.	Protein	9.88

Microbiological Analysis

1.	SPC	16×10^4
2.	SC	28.5×10^3
3.	Coli	No Colony
4.	YMC	No Colony
5.	Pathogens	9.5×10^2

SAMPLE NO. – 10   B/SC

Chemical Analysis

1.	Moisture	9.80
2.	Fat	14.00
3.	Ash	1.9
4.	Sugar	53.37 (17.8 ml)
	(*Bura*)	59.30
5.	Protein	20.93

Microbiological Analysis

1.	SPC	20.5×10^4
2.	SC	34×10^3
3.	Coli	No Colony
4.	YMC	No Colony
5.	Pathogens	7.5×10^2

SAMPLE NO. – 11   P/SC

Chemical Analysis

1.	Moisture	12.60
2.	Fat	22.20
3.	Ash	3.8
4.	Sugar	39.25 (24.2 ml)
	(*Bura*)	43.61
5.	Protein	22.15

Microbiological Analysis

1.	SPC	5×10^4
2.	SC	8×10^3
3.	Coli	No Colony
4.	YMC	No Colony
5.	Pathogens	4×10^2

SAMPLE NO. – 12   P/SC
Chemical Analysis

1.	Moisture	16.20
2.	Fat	24.00
3.	Ash	3.4
4.	Sugar	43.18 (22.0 ml)
	(*Bura*)	47.97
5.	Protein	13.22

Microbiological Analysis

1.	SPC	7.5×10^4
2.	SC	15×10^3
3.	Coli	No Colony
4.	YMC	No Colony
5.	Pathogens	6×10^2

SAMPLE NO. – 13   P/OP
Chemical Analysis

1.	Moisture	10.75
2.	Fat	28.10
3.	Ash	4.1
4.	Sugar	30.15 (31.5 ml)
	(*Bura*)	33.50
5.	Protein	26.90

Microbiological Analysis

1.	SPC	31.5×10^4
2.	SC	111.5×10^3
3.	Coli	No Colony
4.	YMC	No Colony
5.	Pathogens	15×10^2

SAMPLE NO. – 14   P/SC
Chemical Analysis

1.	Moisture	16.00
2.	Fat	19.70
3.	Ash	2.9
4.	Sugar	43.57 (21.8 ml)
	(*Bura*)	48.42
5.	Protein	17.83

Microbiological Analysis

1.	SPC	2×10^4
2.	SC	30.5×10^3
3.	Coli	No Colony
4.	YMC	No Colony
5.	Pathogens	4.5×10^2

SAMPLE NO. – 15   P/SC

Chemical Analysis

1.	Moisture	14.30
2.	Fat	27.20
3.	Ash	3.1
4.	Sugar	26.84 (35.4 ml)
	(*Bura*)	29.81
5.	Protein	28.56

Microbiological Analysis

1.	SPC	17.5×10^4
2.	SC	13.5×10^3
3.	Coli	No Colony
4.	YMC	No Colony
5.	Pathogens	15×10^2

SAMPLE NO. – 16   P/SC

Chemical Analysis

1.	Moisture	11.50
2.	Fat	25.20
3.	Ash	2.5
4.	Sugar	28.61 (32.2 ml)
	(*Bura*)	31.79
5.	Protein	32.19

Microbiological Analysis

1.	SPC	23.0×10^4
2.	SC	26×10^3
3.	Coli	No Colony
4.	YMC	No Colony
5.	Pathogens	18×10^2

SAMPLE NO. – 17   P/SC
Chemical Analysis

1.	Moisture	10.50
1.	Moisture	11.60
2.	Fat	19.20
3.	Ash	1.3
4.	Sugar	51.63 (18.4 ml)
	(*Bura*)	57.37
5.	Protein	16.27

Microbiological Analysis

1.	SPC	39.5×10^4
2.	SC	62×10^3
3.	Coli	No Colony
4.	YMC	No Colony
5.	Pathogens	35×10^2

SAMPLE NO. – 18   P/SC
Chemical Analysis

1.	Moisture	12.40
2.	Fat	27.20
3.	Ash	1.2
4.	Sugar	54.91 (17.3 ml)
	(*Bura*)	61.00
5.	Protein	4.29

Microbiological Analysis

1.	SPC	4×10^4
2.	SC	14×10^3
3.	Coli	No Colony
4.	YMC	No Colony
5.	Pathogens	No Colony

SAMPLE NO. – 19   P/SC
Chemical Analysis

1.	Moisture	17.10
2.	Fat	26.20
3.	Ash	4.8
4.	Sugar	30.65 (31.0 ml)·
	(*Bura*)	34.05
5.	Protein	21.25

Microbiological   Analysis

1.	SPC	17×10^4
2.	SP	16×10^3
3.	Coli	1×10^2
4.	YMC	3×10^2
5.	Pathogens	3×10^2

SAMPLE NO. – 20   P/SC
Chemical Analysis

1.	Moisture	13.20
2.	Fat	18.20
3.	Ash	2.4
4.	Sugar	46.34 (20.5 ml)
	(*Bura*)	51.50
5.	Protein	19.86

Microbiological   Analysis

1.	SPC	24×10^4
2.	SC	37×10^3
3.	Coli	No Colony
4.	YMC	No Colony
5.	Pathogens	2.5×10^2

SAMPLE NO. – 21   P/SC
Chemical Analysis

1.	Moisture	14.00
2.	Fat	19.20
3.	Ash	3.8
4.	Sugar	35.98 (26.4 ml)
	(*Bura*)	39.98
5.	Protein	27.02

Microbiological Analysis

1.	SPC	4×10^4
2.	SC	29×10^3
3.	Coli	No Colony
4.	YMC	No Colony
5.	Pathogens	13×10^2

SAMPLE NO. – 22   L/SC
Chemical Analysis

1.	Moisture	16.35
2.	Fat	21.20
3.	Ash	2.9
4.	Sugar	31.66 (30.0 ml)
	(*Bura*)	35.18
5.	Protein	28.89

Microbiological⁻ Analysis

1.	SPC	21×10^4
2.	SC	43×10^3
3.	Coli	No Colony
4.	YMC	No Colony
5.	Pathogens	17×10^2

SAMPLE NO. – 23   L/SC
Chemical Analysis

1.	Moisture	11.80
2.	Fat	24.00
3.	Ash	2.0
4.	Sugar	24.55 (38.7 ml)
	(*Bura*)	27.27
5.	Protein	37.65

Microbiological Analysis

1.	SPC	6×10^4
2.	SP	21.5×10^3
3.	Coli	No Colony
4.	YMC	No Colony
5.	Pathogens	11×10^2

SAMPLE NO. – 24   L/SC
Chemical Analysis

1.	Moisture	16.00
2.	Fat	28.50
3.	Ash	1.6
4.	Sugar	26.76 (35.5 ml)
	(*Bura*)	29.73
5.	Protein	26.84

Microbiological Analysis

1.	SPC	6×10^4
2.	SP	6×10^3
3.	Coli	No Colony
4.	YMC	No Colony
5.	Pathogens	28×10^2

SAMPLE NO. – 25   L/SC

Chemical Analysis

1.	Moisture	12.80
2.	Fat	34.00
3.	Ash	2.0
4.	Sugar	22.51 (42.2 ml)
	(*Bura*)	25.00
5.	Protein	28.69

Microbiological Analysis

1.	SPC	12×10^4
2.	SC	4×10^3
3.	Coli	No Colony
4.	YMC	No Colony
5.	Pathogens	2×10^2

SAMPLE NO. – 26   L/SC

Chemical Analysis

1.	Moisture	15.60
2.	Fat	27.20
3.	Ash	2.4
4.	Sugar	24.74 (38.4 ml)
	(*Bura*)	27.49
5.	Protein	30.06

Microbiological Analysis

1.	SPC	7.5×10^4
2.	SC	39×10^3
3.	Coli	No Colony
4.	YMC	No Colony
5.	Pathogens	15.5×10^2

SAMPLE NO. – 27   L/SC
Chemical Analysis

1.	Moisture	14.40
2.	Fat	26.00
3.	Ash	1.5
4.	Sugar	23.95 (36.6 ml)
	(*Bura*)	28.84
5.	Protein	32.15

Microbiological Analysis

1.	SPC	18×10^4
2.	SC	44×10^3
3.	Coli	No Colony
4.	YMC	No Colony
5.	Pathogens	40×10^2

SAMPLE NO. – 28   L/SC
Chemical Analysis

1.	Moisture	13.80
2.	Fat	33.60
3.	Ash	1.8
4.	Sugar	23.05 (41.2 ml)
	(*Bura*)	25.62
5.	Protein	27.75

Microbiological Analysis

1.	SPC	15.5×10^4
2.	SC	66×10^3
3.	Coli	No Colony
4.	YMC	No Colony
5.	Pathogens	No Colony

SAMPLE NO. – 29   L/SC
Chemical Analysis

1.	Moisture	17.10
2.	Fat	28.20
3.	Ash	2.1
4.	Sugar	27.46 (34.6 ml)
	(*Bura*)	30.51
5.	Protein	25.14

Microbiological   Analysis

1.	SPC	23.5×10^4
2.	SC	77×10^3
3.	Coli	No Colony
4.	YMC	No Colony
5.	Pathogens	5.5×10^2

SAMPLE NO. – 30   L/SC
Chemical   Analysis

1.	Moisture	15.40
2.	Fat	20.30
3.	Ash	2.4
4.	Sugar	31.88 (29.8 ml)
	(*Bura*)	35.42
5.	Protein	20.02

Microbiological   Analysis

1.	SPC	21.5×10^4
2.	SC	44×10^3
3.	Coli	No Colony
4.	YMC	No Colony
5.	Pathogens	9×10^2

PREPARATION OF SOLUTIONS

Preparation of standard reagent, Indicators solution and media used for the analysis of *burfi*, *peda* and *lodge* in this study.

1. HCl 60 per cent

Sixty ml HC1 (100%) was added to 40 ml of distilled water.

2. NaOH 5 per cent

Weighed 5 grams of NaOH sticks in a beaker and immediately dissolved in 100 ml of distilled water.

3. Fehling Solution

Solution A : 34.693 g $CuSO_4$. $5H_2O$ was dissolved in 500 ml of distilled water.
Solution B : 173 g Rochelle salt and 50 grams Caustic soda (KOH) were dissolved in 500 ml/distilled water.
Equal volume of both the solution (A and B) were mixed immediately before use.

4. Co-effier's Methylene Blue

One gram of methylene blue was added to 100 ml of distilled water.

5. N/9 NaOH

Four thousand and nineteen grams of NaOH were dissolved in 1000 ml of distilled water and the solution was standardized with N/9 Oxalic acid using Phenolphthalein as an indicator.

6. Lactic acid 10 per cent

10 ml Lactic acid (100 per cent pure) was added to 90 ml distilled water.

7. Physiological Normal saline solution

Nine grams of chemically pure sodium chloride (NaCl) was dissolved in 1000 ml of distilled water and solution was distributed in test tubes and conical flasks in required quantities. These test tubes and conical flasks sterilized in autoclave at 15 lbs psi for 20 minutes.

8. Standard milk Agar

Composition

Peptone	5 g
Yeast Extract	3 g
Milk/Glucose	10 g
Distilled water	1000 ml
pH	6.8
Agar-Agar	16 g

Ingredients were dissolved in distilled water by heating to 100°C the contents were cooled and the pH was adjusted to 6.8. In a separate beaker Agar-Agar was dissolved in 500 ml distilled water and the contents auto-clave at 15 lbs for 5 minutes. The pH adjusted broth and the Agar-Agar was mixed together and tubing was done in 1 ml quantities. The tubes were auto-claved at 15 lbs psi for 20 minutes.

9. Nutrient gas

Composition

Peptone	10 g
NaCl	5 g
Lab Camce	10 g
Distilled water	1000 ml
Agar-Agar	16 g
pH	7.2

The ingredients were dissolved in distilled water by heating to 100°C. The contents were cooled ad the pH was adjusted to 7.2. In a separate beaker agar-agar was dissolved in 500 ml distilled water and the contents were autoclaved at 15 lbs psi for 5 minutes.

The pH adjusted broth and the agar-agar were mixed together and tubing was done. The tobes were autoclaved at 15 lbs psi for 20 minutes.

10. Violet Red Bile Salt Agar

Composition

Peptone	7.0 g
Yeast extract	3.0 g
Bile extract (Sodium Tarochelate)	1.5 g
Sodium Chloride	5.0 g
Lactose	10.0 g
Neutral red	0.03 g
Crystal Violet	0.0002 g
Agar-Agar	15.0 g
Distilled water	1000 ml
pH	7.4

Peptone, Yeast Extract, bile salt and sodium chloride were dissolved in distilled water at 100°C. The broth was adjusted at pH 7.4. In a separate beaker Agar-Agar was dissolved in 500 ml. Distilled water. Lactose, neutral red and crystal violet were added and mixed untill dissolved. Tubing was done the tubes were sterilised in auto-clave 15 lbs psi for 20 minutes.

11. Potato Deatrose Agar :

Composition

Potato (Peeled and dried)	200 g
D-Glucose	20 g
Agar-Agar	15 g
Distilled water	1000 ml

Boiled 200 g peeled, dried and sliced potato in one litre water for about one hour the contents were filtered through a fine musline cloth and the volume of the filtrate was made up to one litre by distilled water. Finally glucose and agar-agar were added to the broth. The medium was distributed in tubes and sterilised 15 lbs psi minutes. pH was adjusted at the time of puring with the help of 10 per cent Lactic acid.

12. Staphylococcus medium – 110

Composition

Tryptone	10.0 g
Yeast Extract	2.5 g
Sodium Chloride	75.0 g
a – Mannitol	10.0 g
Lactose	2.0 g
Gelatin	30.0 g
Depotassium phosphate	5.0 g
Agar	15.0 g
Distilled water	1000 ml
pH	6.0

Tryptone yeast extract, sodium chloride and dipotassium phosphate were dissolved in 500 ml distilled water at 100°C. The broth was adjusted at pH 6.0. In a separate beaker agar-agar was dissolved in 500 ml distilled water. Lactose a-mannitol and gelatin were added to broth after adjustment of pH and mixed until dissolved. The broth and agar-agar were mixed together and 10 ml quantities of this agar-medium was filled in test tubes. These test tubes were sterilised in autoclave at 15 lbs psi for 20 minutes.

BIBLIOGRAPHY

Adhikari, A.K., Mathur, O. N. and Patil G.R. (1993). "Development of microstructure in acid and heat coagulated Indegenous milk products". "Indian Journals of Dairy Sc." 46(10): 477-482.

Adhikari, A.K., Mathur, O.N. and Patil G.R. (1994). Inter relationship among Instron textural parameters composition and microstructure of *Khoa* and *guilabjamun* made from buffalo milk. J food se and techno. 31(4): 279-284.

Arora, K.L., Harish Chander and Jessa Ram (1991). "Chemical and microbiological quality of *Kalakhand* sold in market" Asian Dairy 10(2): 96-102.

Bautista, E.S., Dahiya, R.S. and Speck, M.L. (1966) Identification of Compounds Causing symbiotic growth of *Str. thermophilus* and *Lac. Bulgaricus* in milk". J. Dairy Res., 33: 299.

Bills, D.D., Scanla, R.C., Lindsay, R.C. and Sather, L. (1972). "Effects of Sucrose on the Production of Acetaldeyde acids by Yoghurt Culture Bacteria". J. Dairy Sci. 55(11), 1570-73.

Boatazzi, V. and Delluglio, F. (1967) Acetaladehyde and diacetyl Production by *Str. thermophilous* and other lactic Streptococci.

Boghra, V.R. and Mathur, O.M. (1991). "Chemical quality of some marketed Indigenous milk product". Journal of food Sc. And Tech. 28(1): 59-60.

Bottazzi, V. and Vescova, M. (1969). "Carbonyl compounds produced by Yoghurt Bacteria". Neth Milk Dairy J. 23: 71.

Braz, M. and Allen, L.A. (1938). "Protein Metabolism and Acid Production by the lactic Acid and bacteria in milk Influence of Yeast Extract and chalk". J. Dairy Res. 10: 20.

Bull, M.E. (1947). Studies on milk proteins II colorimotric Determination of the Partial Hydrolysis of the Proteins in milk.

Bundgaard, A.G., Olsen, O.J. and Madnen, R.F. (1972). Ultrafiltration and Hyperfilteration of Skim milk of production of various Dairy Production". Dairy Ind. 37: 539.
by *Str. thermophilus*". Noth. Milk Dairy J. 22: 50.

Cowman, R.A. and Speak, M.L., (1962). "Activity of lactics trept. ococci Following Ultra low tempertaure Storage". J. Dairy Sci 49(5): 609.

Cowman, R.A. and Speek, M.L. (1963). "Reduction in Proteolytic Activity at Low temperature". J. App. Microbiol 15: 851.

Crawford, R.J.M. (1962). "How to succeed wit. Yoghurt". Dairy Eng. 79(1): 4.

Crawford, R.J.M. (1975). "Residencial course on short shelf life Dairy Products". J. Soc. Dairy Bacterial.

Crudzinskaya, E.E. and Koroleva, N.S. (1970). "Changen in Amino Acid Spectrum. Inst. Moloch." Prom., 27: 63.

Date, W.B. and Bhattia, D.S. (1955) "Preservation of Indian milk sweets-some preliminary studies on Shrikand wodi and milk *burfi*", Indian J. Dairy Sci., 8(2): 61-66.

Dav, R.I. and Shah N.P. (1996). "Evaluation of media for selective Enumeration of Streptococcus, thermophilus, lactobacillus debruckii S and P, bulgaricus Lactobacillus acidophilus and bifido bacteria." J Dairy Sc. 79(9): 1529-1536.

Davis, F.L., Shanker, P.A. and Underwood, H.M. (1977). "The use of Milk concentrated by Reverse Osmosis for the Manufaccture of Yoghurt". J. Soc. Dairy Technol. 30(1): 23-25

Davis, J.G. (1956). "Yoghurt and other Cutured Milks". J.Soc. Dairy Technol. 9: 69 (117, 160)

Davis, J.G. (1971). "Enumeration and Viability of *L. bulgaricus* and *Str. thermophilus* in Yoghurts". Dairy Ind. 36(10): 569.

Davis, J.G. (1973). "Yoghurt Manufacture". Food Manufacture, 48 : 23.

Donnlly, J.K., O'Sullivan, A.C. and Deleney, R.A.M. (1974). "Reversee Osmosis – concentration Applications". J. Soc. Dairy Technol. 27: 128.

Dutta, S.M., Kuila, R.K., Arora, B.C. and Ranganathan, B. (1972). "Effect of Indubation temperature on acid and Falvour Production in milk by Lactic Acid bacteria". J. Milk and Food Technol. 35(4): 242-244.

Dutta, S.M., Kuila, R.K., Ranganathan, B. and Laxminarayana, H. (1971a). "Biochemical changes Produced by in milk by Selected Cultures of Lactic acid bacteria". Ind. J. Dairy Sci. 24: 107.

Dutta, S.M., Kuila, R.K., Ranganathan, B. and Laxminarayana, H. (1971b). "A comparative study of the activity of starter culturese in different types of milk". Milchwissenschaft 26: 158-161.

Dwarkanath, C.T. and Srikanta, S. (1997). "Studies on the microbiological quality of traditional Indian sweet-meet products." J. FD. Sci, and Tech., 14(5): 201-203.

Egli, F. and Egli, G. (1977). "Process for the Production of Sterile

Formisano, M., Percuoco, G. and Percuoco, S. (1970). "Proteolytic Activity of Yoghurt Starters", Industrie Agrarie II, 3.

Galesloot, Th.E. (1962). "The Bacteriology and Biochemistry of Starter and Ripened Cream". XVI Int. Dairy Congr D, 143-159.

Galesloot, Th.E., Hassing, F. and Veringa, H.D. (1961). "Agar Media Voor Het I Soleren En Tollon Van Aroma Bacterien In Zuursols Neth". Milk Dairy J. 15: 127.

Galesloot, Th.E., Hassing, F. and Veringa, H.D. (1968). "Symbiosis in Yoghurt Stimulation of *Lac. Bulgaricus* by a factor produced

Garg, S.R. ; Usha, V. and Mondokhot (1984). "Studies on microbial and chemical profile of some Indian sweetmeats and their significance". Indian J. Dairy Sci., 37(4): 332-333.

Gatler, W.N., Fermades. Y. and Sant, M.V. (1970). "Bacteria From Sweatmeat of Bombay." Indian J. Dairy microbiology, 10(3): 65-68.

Ghodekar, D.R.: Dudani, A.T. and Ranganathan (1974). "Microbiological quality of Indian Milk Products". J. Milk Fd. Tech., 37(3): 119-122.

Ghodekar, D.R. (1969). M.Sc. Thesis, Bombay Uni., Bombay.

Ghodeker, D.R., Raganathan, B. and Dudani, A.T. (1980). "Yeasts and Moulds in Indigenous milk products". Indian J. Dairy Sci., 33(2): 255-256.

Gilliland and Olson (1963). "Acid Production". J. Dairy Sci. 46(6): 609.

Gorner, F., Palo, V., and Bertanova, M. (1968)., "Veranderunge des Gehaltes der Fluchtigen Stoffe Wahrondder Joghurtrol Fung" Milchwissenschaft 23(2): 94.

Goyal, G.K. and Srinivasan, M.R. (1989). "Effect of packaging on the chemical quality of *Khoa* during storage. Indian Dairy Sci 42(2): 165-170.

Hamevathy J., Rananna. B.R. and Potty, V.H. (1974) "Studies on commercial *burfi* proparetions some preliminary observations." Indian food Packer. 28(3): 29-30.

Harvey, R.J. (1960). "Production of Acetone and acetaldehyde By Lactic Streptococci". J. Dairy Res., 27: 41.

Hary and Jackson, H. (1967). "Preparation of Soyabean cheese using

Hawley, H.B. (1957). "Methods in Food Technology". Food Manufactuae. 32: 370.

Hempenius, W.L. (1968). "Methods for determining Volatile Acids in culture Dairy Products". J. Dairy Sci. 51: 221.

Henry, R.J. (1972). "Effect of Oxygen on glucose Dissimi-Lation by Heterolac bactria". J. Gen. Appl. Microbiol. 23: 1153.

Higashio, K., Kikuchi, T. and Furuichi, E. (1978). "The Symbiosis between *Lac. bulgaricaus* and *Str. thermophilus* in Yoghurt Cultures". XX Int. Dairy Congr., Paris, p. 515.

Humphrey, C.L. and Plunkett, M. (1969). Yoghurt: A Review of its manufacture. Dairy Sci. Abstr. *31*(11): 607-622.

I.S.I. (1962). "Bacteriological Tests of milk." I.S.I (1979), Manak Bhawan, New Delhi.

Indian Standards Institution (1960). Methods of Test for Dairy Ind (Part I) Rapid Examination of milk (Part II); IS: (1979).

Iyngar, M.K.K., Nambudripad, V.K.N. and Dadani, A.T. (1967). Effect of Heat Treatment of Buffalo and Cow milk in the manufacture of Yoghurt. Ind. J. Dairy Sci. *20*: 8.

Jadhav, N.S., Waghmare, P.S. and Zanjad, P.N. (1990) "Observation on the dehydration of heat Induced milk foam for *khoa* making". Indian J Dairy Sci. *43*(2) 185-189.

Jap.J., Zootech., Sci 29(6): 632.

Jatkar, S., Sharda D., and Rajalaxmi (1984). "Microbiological quality of market milk sweets in twin cities Hyderabad and Secunderabad." Dairy Sci Abstracts 46(10): 764.

Johannsen, G.B. (1975). Starter Cultures Dairy Sci. Abstr. 37(1): 337.

Jonsson, H. and Petterson, H.E. (1977). Aroma Formation in Lactic Starter Cultures Nordish Mejeriindustri 4 (5): 241, 245-257, Cited from Dairy Sci. Abstr. (1977) 39: 12.

Kamat, M.Y. and Sulebele, G.A. (1974). "Microbiological quality of *Peda*. "J.Fd. Sci. and Tech., *11*(2): 50-51.

Kanwar, J.S. and Chopra, S.L. (1959). "Practical agricultural Chemistry". S. Chand and Co., New Delhi.

Keenan, T.W. and Bills, D.D (1968). The influence of Lacto-bacilli on Open Texture in Cheddar Cheese. N. Zealand J. Dairy Tech. 7: 159-160.

Kicrmeir, F. (1972). The use of Fruit for Dairy Products. Cited from Dairy Sci. Abstr. *35*(4): 1132.

Kim, C.S. and Shin H.S. (1971). Studies on the Preparation of a cheese likeproduct from soyabean milk. Dairy Sci. Abstr. *33*: 82.

Kohl, H. (1976). Technical measures for the Improvement of the keeping quality of fresh milk Product, Particularly cultured milk products. Cited from Dairy Sci. Abstr. 39(1): 119.

Kon, S.K. (1959). Differentation between the traditional Yoghurt and cultured yoghurt. FAO Nutrition study no. 17.

Kudchodkar, B.G and Singh, I.P. (1964). "Incidence of Enterotexogenic type staphylococci in indigenous milk products," Indian. J. Dairy Sci., 17(4): 144.

Kulshrestha, S.B. (1978), "Occurrence of Salmonella in milk products." Indian J.Dairy Sci., 31: 381.

Kumar, B., Das, S. and Sawhhey, I.K. (1990) "Development of self life simulation model for *khoa*" Aabstract Brief Communication of the XXIII International Dairy Congress Montreal Oct. 8 vol. II, p. 449.

Kurmann, J. (1966). Effect of storage temperature on Yoghurt mother culture. Dairy Sci. Astr. 28: 458.

Lactic starter Organisms". J. Food Technol. 21: 95-97.

Lang, F. and Lang, A. (1973). Progress in the Mechanisation, Packaging and Extension of keeping quality of Yoghurt Milk Ind. 73(3-4): 17-18, 28-30, 33.

Lavania, G.S., and Gautam, S.N. (1987). "Microbiological quality of sweets made out of *khoa*." Dairy Guide 9(3): 29.

Laxminarayana, H., Nambudripad, V.K.N. Laxminarayana, V., Ananlharamlah, S.N. Sreenivasamuthy, V., and Iya, K.K. (1952). Studies on *Dahi* Taxonomy of the Lactic Acid Bacteria of *Dahi*. Int. J. Vety. Sci. and Anti. Husb. 22 (1): 27-49.

Lee, G.J. and Jago, C.R. (1977). Formation of Acetaldehyde from 2-deoxy D-Ribose, 5 Phosphate in Lactic Acid Bactria. J. Dairy Res. 44 (1): 139-144.

Lee, J.S. and Price, R.J. (1969). Inhibition of Food Spoilage Organisms. Bact. Proc. 13.

Lee, S.Y. Vedamuthu, (1974). An Agar Medium for the Differential and enumeration of Yoghurt Starter bactria. J. Dairy Sci. 44: 807.

Lindsay, C., Day, E.A. and Sadine, W.E. (1965). Rapid Quantitative Method for Determination of Acetal-dehyde in Lactic Starter cultures. J. Dairy Sci. 48: 665.

Lindsay, R.C., Day, E.A. and Sadine, W.E. (1965). Green flavour defect in Lactic starter cultures J. Dairy Sci. 48: 863-869.

Luca, C. (1974). Effect of repreated drying and ultra Viloet irradiation on Lactic Acid Bacteria Industrial Alimentaria 25(6): 291-293

Mabbit, L.A. (1961). Review of the Progress of Dairy Science Flavour of cheedar cheese. J. Dariy Res. 28: 293, 303.

Magadum, R.B., Anatakrishnan, C.P. and Natrajan, A.M. (1988) "Chemical and *bacteriological quality* of market sample of *Kalakand.*" Cherison. 17(5): 200-201.

Maksimova, A.K. (1968). Intensified Production of cultured Milk products. Moloch. Prom. 29(9): 212 Cited from Dairy Sci. Abstr. 31 429.

Mandokhot, V.V. and Garg, S.R. (1985). "Market quality of *Khoa, burfi* and *peda* A critical review". J. Fd. Sci and Tech., 22(4): 299-303.

Marth, E.H. (1962). Certain Aspects of Starter culture Metabolism

Miller, I. and Kandler, O. (1964). Das Aminosaurespektrum Von Joghurt. Milchwissenschaft. 19(1): 18.

Miyani, R.V. and Vyas, S.H. (1990) "Rheological properties of *khoa* as influenced by acidity of milk" (Dairy Sci abstract) 521.

Mocquot, G. and Hurrel, C. (1970). The Selection and use of Som micro-orgs for the manufacture of fermented and adidifeod milk products. J. Soc. Dairy Technol. 23: 130.

Moona, Nancy, J. and Reinbold, G.W. (1976). Commensalism and competition in mixed cultures of *Lac. bulgaricus* and *Str. thermophilus.* J. Milk Food Techno. 39(5): 337-341.

Mulay, C.A. and Lodkani, B.G (1973). "Comparative assessment of quality of *khoa* and their products from homogenized and unhomogenized milk." J.Fd. Sci Tech., 10: 110.

Nachev, L. (1969). Future trends in Food Processing and Marketing Dairy Sci. Abstr. 29: 1220.

Naylor, J. and Sharpe, M.E. (1958). Lactobacilli in choddar cheese.

Neiricuckz (1972). Thermisation of Yoghurt. Dairy Ind, 37: 274.

Pack, M.Y., Sandine, E.R. and Day, E.A. (1964) Diacetyl Production and destruction Patterns in mixed strain starter cultures. J. Dairy Sci. 47: 674.

Padake, N.Y., Gholap, A.S. and Subblakshmi, G. (1994) "Essential iol of Decalepis hamiltonii as an antimicrobial agent", J. of Food Sci and Tech. 31(6): 472-475.

Patel, A.A., Patil, G.R., Garg, F.C. and Gupta, S.K. (1992) Effect of concentration condition on texture of *khoa.*

Patel, G.G. (1985). "Becteriological quality of *Peda* and *burfi* with special reference to certain bacteries of Public health significante", J. Fd. Sci and Tech., 22(3): 133.

Patel, M.M. (1986) "A study in *Penda* manaufacture", Indian Dairyman: 38(5): 253.

Pette, J.W, and Lolkema, H. (1950a). Symbiose En Antibiose in Mengcultures Van L.B. bulgaricus EN SC. Thermophilus. Neth. Milk Dairy J. 4: 197-208.

Pette, J.W, and Lolkema, H. (1950b). ZUURVORMING EN Aroma Vorming in Yoghurt.

Prajapati, P.S., Thakar, P.N., Miyani, R.V. and Upadhyay, K.G. (1990) "Influence of use of *khoa* prepared from concentrated milk kon quality of *Gulabjamun*". Abstract, October 8-12 Vol. II 530.

Rajorhia, G.S; and Sen, D.C. (1987) "Problems of milk sweets made in India". Indian Dairyman, 39(6): 283-285.

Rajoria, G.S., Pal, D. and Garg, F.C. (1991) "Evaluation of the *quality of khoa* prepared from different Machanised System." Indian J. Dairy Sci. 44(2): 181-187.

Rakshy, S.E.S.E. (1966). Der Erhitzungseffect bei der Pasteuri Sierung von Johurt and Sauermilch.

Ramanna, B.R., Bhat, K.K., Mahadeveiah, B., Dwarkananth, C.T., Dhanaraj, S., Potty, V.H. and Sen (1983). "Investigations on lerge scale preparation and Preservations of milk *burfi*." J.Fd Sci. and Tech, 20(1): 67-70.

Ranganathan, B. (1984). "Market qualtiy of Dairy products" Indian Dairyman 36(12): 66.

Rasic, J. and Milanovic, S. (1966). Diacetyl Production Le Lait 428: 489.

Rasic, J., Stajsavljeviz T. and Curcic, R. (1971). A study on the amono acids of Yoghurt II Amino acids content and biological value of the Proteins of different kinds of Yoghurt. Milchwissenschaft 26: 29.

Reddy, C.R. and Rajorhia, G.S. (1992): "Present status of *peda* and *burfi* technology a Review", Indian J. Dairy Sci 45(5): 220-225.

Reddy, C.S. and Datta, A.K. (1994) "Thermophysical properties of Reconstituted milk during processing", J. Food Engineering, 21(1): 31-40.

Reddy, V.P. and Khan, M.M.H. (1993) "Effect of antimicrobial agents and packaging materials on the *microbial quality* of *khoa*". J. Food Sci and Tech. 30(2): 130-131.

Research Notes (1975). "Enterotoxigenecity and phage typing of Stayphylococcal isolated from *peda*". Indian Fd. Sci & Tech., 12 (6): 316.

Robinson, R.K. (1977). Acetaldehyde as an Indicator of Flavour Intensity in Yoghurt. Milk Ind. 79(4): 4-6.

Robinson, R.K. and Tamime, A.Y. (1976). Quality Appraisal of Yoghurt. J. Soc. Dairy Technol. 29: 148.

Robinson, R.K. and Tamimi , A.Y. (1975). Yoghurt – A Review of the Product and its manufacture. J. Soc. Dairy Technol. 28 (3): 149.

Rogosa, M., Mitchell, A.W. and Ralph F. Wiseman (1951) A selective medium for the Isolation and Enumeration of oral and fecal Lactobacilli. J. Bacteriol. 62: 132.

Roiner, F.X.J. and Grosserhode, J. (1972). Method for Producing cultured milk Products Cited from Dairy Sci. Abstr. 34(8): 3573.

Sachadeva, S. and Rajorhia, G.S. (1982). "Technology and shelf life of *Burfi*." Indian J. Dairy Sci. 35(4), 513.

Sapre, M. and Deodhas, A.D. (1991). "Effect of *khoa* prepration from buffalo milk on protein quality", Indian J. Dairy Sci 44(10), 624-628.

Sasaki, R. and Nakae, T. (1958). Determination of Proteolytic Activity

Sasaki, R. and Nakae, T. (1959). Proteolytic Activity of Lactic acid Bacteria. Jap. J., Zootech Sci 30(1): 7

Schulz, M..E. and Thingst, G. (1954). Cotorimetric determination of acctaldehyde in Yoghurt. Milchwissenschaft 9: 330.

Searles, M.A., Argyle, P.J., Chandan, R. and Gordon, J.E. (1970) Lipolytic and Proteolytic Activity of Lactic cultures. X, VIII Int. Dairy Congr. IE, 111.

Seneca, I., Henderion, E. and Collins, A. (1950). Acetaldhyde – Principal Flavour component of Yoghurt. Am. Practur Dig. Trent 1: 1252.

Shanker, P.A. and Davis, F.L. (1978). Inter-relationships of *Str. Thermophilus* and *Lac. bulgaricus* in Yoghurt Starters.

Sharma, U.P. and Zariwala, I.T. (1978). "Survey of quality of milk products in Bombay." J.Fd Sci and Tech. 15(3), 118-121

Singh, J. and Ranganathan B. (1978). A comparison of the Activity *Lac. bulgaricus* and one of its mutants in Different types of milk. J.D.R. (45): 123-125

Singh, K.., Ogra, J.L. and Rai, Y.S. (1975). "Survey of Microbiological quality of *burfi* and *peda* in Allahabad." Indian J. Dairy Sci., 28 (3), 219-220.

Singh, S. and Rao, K.H. (1992). "Goat milk product technology A Review." Indian J. Dairy Sci 45; (1) 572-587.

Speckmann, R.A. and Collins E.B. (1968). Diacetyl Biosynthesis in *Streptococcus diacetilactis* and *Leuconostoc cirtrovorum* J.Bacteriol. 95: 174.

Srinivasan, L.M. (2001). *Microbiology*, Shree Publishers, New Delhi.

Srinivasan, M.R. and Goyal, G.K. (1989). "Influence on the water vapur transmission rate of flexible package during storage of *Khoa*." Chairon 18(3), 129-131.

Srinivasan, M.R. and Rajorhia, G.S. (1976). "The case of *khoa* for a rightful place among dairy products." Indian Dairyman, 28(1), 11.

Tamine, A.Y. and Robinson, R.K. (1976). Yoghurt – Science and Technology. Diary Ind. Int. 41(11): 408-411.

Teply, M. (1970). Some Recent Technical Advance and Probable Trends in Processing, Manufacture and Packaging of New Dairy Foods. XVIII, Int.: Dairy Cognr. 1E: 404.

Terkazaryan, S. (1974). Formation of Volatile fatty acids by different Species of lactic acid bacteria from various sources. Diary Sci. Abstract 36(2).

Thomas, K.S., (1966). Comparative Studies on the Growth and Bio-chemical Activities of Starter organisms in Cow and Buffalo Milk. XVIII Int. Dairy Congr. D., 2, 455.

Tramer, J. (1973). Yoghurt Cultures Nature 211: 204.

Varadaraja, M.C., Madev, B.S. and Ashfaq, Ahmad (1983). "Staphylocci in Indian milk products as potential Health Hazards." Indian Dairyman 35(5), 301.

Veringa, H.A. and Galenroot, Th.E. (1968) Symbiosis in Youghurt III Isolation and Indentification of a growth factor for *Lactobacillus bulgariucs* Produced by *Streptococcus thermophilus* Neth. Milk Dairy J. 22: 114 - 120.

Vijayabhader and Kalpana, Y. Patel (1983), "Composition and Packaging of Pedha." Indian J. Dairy Sci, 36(2), 187-192.

Viyas, S.H and Miyani, R.Y. (1990). "Impact of Sodiumcitrate addition to milk on textural and Sensory quality of *Khoa*." (Dairy Sci abstract). Oct 8-12, Vol. II 520.

www.ingramcontent.com/pod-product-compliance
Lightning Source LLC
Chambersburg PA
CBHW070709190326
41458CB00004B/918